Learn to Read Chinese

An Introduction to the Language and Concepts of Current *Zhongyi* Literature

by

Paul U. Unschuld

Volume One

Texts, Transcription, Vocabulary, Translations

Paradigm Publications
Brookline, Massachusetts, 1994

Software by Rupprecht Mayer
Electronic Layout by Anton Lachner

Library of Congress Cataloging in Publication Data

Unschuld, Paul U. (Paul Ulrich), 1943-
[Chinesisch lesen lernen. English]
Learn To Read Chinese : an introduction to the language and concepts of current Zhongyi literature / by Paul U. Unschuld.
p. cm.
Includes bibliographical references and index.
ISBN 0-912111-46-1 (v. 1) : $ 30.00. -- ISBN 0-912111-47-X (v. 2) : $ 30.00
1. Chinese language--Readers--Medicine, Chinese. 2. Medicine, Chinese. I. Title.
PL1117.5.M43U4713 1994
495.1'86421'02461--dc20
94-16448
CIP

Paradigm Publications 44 Linden Street, Brookline, Massachusetts 02146 U.S.A.

Printed in the Unites States of America

LEARN TO READ CHINESE

Volume One

CONTENTS

Preface

This primer is for anyone seeking direct linguistic access to contemporary Chinese technical literature. Although companion audio tapes are available, the title emphasizes reading Chinese because the text offers no exercises in conversation. Rather it provides a complete system for acquiring familiarity with and comprehension of contemporary [Chinese-language] literature on traditional Chinese medicine. However, *Learn to Read Chinese* is grounded in a new didactic approach known as "natural language development" that makes it a suitable course of instruction for any broader, more general study of Chinese technical writing.

Chinese medicine was chosen as a didactic focus because in recent decades the number of persons who require the ability to read and understand its technical literature has grown so dramatically. The text source selected serves this need. All 128 of the texts that form the sixteen lessons of this primer are quotations from the ninth edition of *Zhongyi rumen* ("Introduction to Chinese Medicine") by Qin Bowei.[1] This gives those who seek facility with technical medical literature the opportunity to immediately focus on contemporary *zhongyi* texts, that is, the literature of contemporary Chinese medicine.

Until now, practice with *zhongyi* texts has required a year or two of intensive study of general, lay Chinese. Because no appropriate textbook existed, a necessary level of linguistic competence had to be reached before the ability to read *zhongyi* literature could be acquired. However, beginning with the first lesson of *Learn to Read Chinese* readers receive the technical vocabulary and information required to pursue their aim.

The program consists of two volumes. The first contains sixteen lessons each of which includes eight short texts. All of these 128 texts are presented in Chinese characters, pinyin transcription, and English translation. Each text is followed by a cumulative vocabulary. Beginning with Lesson One, each vocabulary list contains every newly-introduced

---

[1] Qin Bowei 秦伯未, *Zhongyi rumen* 中医入门, Ninth edition, People's Hygiene Publishing Company, Peking, 1981.

character. These lists also contain previously introduced characters that appear in a second or third meaning. Everywhere the pinyin transcriptions of Chinese characters contain the five tone marks that clarify pronunciation. Where necessary for understanding the concepts contained in these text, short explanatory notes have been added.

The lessons follow a thematic order, first offering an introduction to the concepts of traditional Chinese medicine. Regardless, until students reach the degree of skill required to appreciate the detail of contemporary or historic Chinese medical concepts directly from Chinese texts, they should view this volume as a guide to language and consult appropriate English secondary literature as needed. My book *Medicine in China, A History of Ideas*[2] surveys the historical development of concepts of health and illness in China and may help explain the concepts referenced.

Readers should keep in mind that the texts collected in this primer were written by a contemporary author and read by contemporary Chinese audiences based on a shared knowledge of modern scientific anatomy, physiology, and etiology. The translation of these texts into English must account for this intellectual environment. Thus there are technical terms that have assumed meanings different from those they carried in earlier centuries. Concepts such as "organs" or "organism" for example were never part of traditional Chinese understanding of the human body. However, today, they are frequently used by modern writers and practitioners of traditional Chinese medicine. Students who wish to supplement their study of *Learn to Read Chinese* by becoming familiar with the origin and use of ancient Chinese medical terms in primary sources should consult my text *Introductory Readings in Classical Chinese Medicine*.[3]

The specific didactic innovations of this textbook are realized in Volume Two. All 64 texts of the first eight lessons in Volume One are presented as what I have named "structural units." This is an analysis that does not impose Latin syntactic notations on the Chinese language. This system

---

[2] Paul U.Unschuld, *Medicine in China. A History of Ideas*, University of California Press, Berkeley, CA, 1985.

[3] Paul U.Unschuld, *Introductory Readings in Classical Chinese Medicine*, Kluwer Academic Publishers, Dordrecht, Netherlands, 1988.

permits the student to trace the translation of every statement from the original Chinese text to its appropriate translation. For example, the English translations in Volume One have been rendered as close as is possible to the structure of the Chinese text. However, because the stylistic requirements of the English language differ from those of Chinese, each sentence has acquired a certain distance from the original. By presenting the original sentences as structural units, this distance is bridged and the process of translation made apparent.

By "sentences" I mean the entire statement expressed between periods. The structure of Chinese sentences rarely parallels English sentences. Some Chinese sentences may consist of only one statement the structure of which is comparable to an English sentence. However, in general, Chinese technical prose is composed of lengthy structures that link two or more statements into a single sentence. It is not, for example, unusual for the subject to change in each statement of a lengthy structure. Thus in Volume Two each complex sentence is parsed as one "Basic Statement" and one or more "Adjunct Statements." The isolation of Basic and Adjunct Statements is the first major step in making the text transparent to the reader.

The separation of Basic and Adjunct Statements is reinforced by presenting each in a graphic frame that isolates the Chinese characters and transliteration. Through this emphasis and the continuous repetition of the structural units, the reader learns to differentiate what once appeared to be only an amorphous cluster of characters. Because the use of the unchanging pictograms is not revealed by declination or conjugation, or as a substantive a verb, adverb or adjective, or even as a grammatical particle, it is structure that best informs. Thus each structural unit is, where possible, further differentiated into what I have called a "Key Statement" and its modifications.

In general, but not always, a Key Statement is comparable to the English sentence structure of subject – verb – object. However, a Key Statement may sometimes be reduced to a single verb, the subject of which must be remembered from a previous statement, or be inferred from the context. Through parallel presentation of Chinese characters, their pinyin transliteration and literal translation, students become able to identify each Key

Statement in a lengthy chain of characters, whether it is part of a Basic or Adjunct Statement. Students are thus also able to trace how the English translation given in Volume One was derived from the original Chinese text.

An excellent example of how an awareness of structure helps is Chinese bracket phrases. These phrases are composed of two or three characters that are positioned separately in a sentence. These often appear at the beginning and ending of a statement thus "bracketing" a particular notion. The first example of this is to be found in Lesson 1.3 where the Chinese expression *zài ... fāng-miàn* corresponds to English uses "as for ..." or "in regard to." So too *yòng ... lái* corresponds to "with" and *zài ... shàng* corresponds to both "in" and "as far as ... is concerned." In the absence of declination and conjugation, bracket phrases assume an important grammatical function by delineating the structure of a sentence. Thus these phrases are emboldend to help readers learn to search for them when attempting to decipher lengthy statements.

What I referred to earlier as "modifications" are often adverbial, adjective or genitive structures used to modify the subjects, verbs, or objects within a statement. Identifying such modifiers in a complex Chinese sentence structure is one of the more difficult tasks a beginning reader must face. In addition to the break-down of sentences and statements into structural units presented in Volume Two, these modifiers are pointed out through a simple pattern of questions and answers. Thus students learn to recognize modifications as structural units, separate them from Key Statements, and adequately translate them.

Natural Language Development applies the methods of learning that are used by children who are born into a mature linguistic environment. While adults may occasionally use only the most simple structures when speaking to children, from the child's perspective he or she is slowly learning to make sense of the complex sentences used by adults. Children first learn key terms and key statements isolating them from complex sentences. Next they learn to identify modifications of these key terms and statements. Only in a third and final stage do they become able to link key statements and adjunct statements. Similar principles guide a student using these textbooks toward a mastery of technical Chinese. In contrast to common primers, *Learn to Read Chinese* does not begin with artificially simplified sentences, progressing lesson by lesson toward meaningful expression. Instead, students immediately begin with actual technical prose as the didactic approach of Volume Two guides them from linguistic childhood to maturity.

These textbooks are thus suited for beginners as well as those who have already acquired an advanced mastery of lay Chinese. By studying these sixteen lessons advanced students will quickly expand their expertise and learn the special vocabulary and diction of *zhongyi* literature. However, the main group of students expected to use of these textbooks are beginning students who will work through these primers with or without the aid of a teacher. For self-teaching, the Chinese characters of the first four lessons are explained in a stroke-order list that contains all possible stroke orders needed to write a character or count its strokes. Thus they will learn to use dictionaries that are based on stroke count. Furthermore, tapes of all sixteen lessons are available to assist learning the proper pronunciation and reading of the texts.

Volume Two concludes with a general glossary of all characters and their meanings as they appear in the original texts of Volume One (ordered alphabetically on the basis of their pinyin transliteration). This general glossary is a useful dictionary for recalling the meaning of characters that were introduced in earlier lessons. The pronunciation of unknown characters can also be known through the pinyin transliteration of each short text that is presented in Volume One. This allows for finding the character, the previously-introduced meanings, and a reference to its earlier appearance in the general glossary.

This primer is an adapted English version of the original German edition. I am most grateful to Nigel Wiseman for reading the manuscript and offering many valuable suggestions aimed toward our common goal of an increasing standardization of English translations of Chinese *zhongyi* literature on a philological level that does justice to both the historical and modern context of its terminology.

Munich, March 1994 Paul U. Unschuld

LESSON 1: THE YINYANG DOCTRINE

Text 1.1

中医用阴阳学说来说明医学上的基本问题，从而成为中医理论的思想体系，它贯串在中医学中的生理，病理，诊断，治疗和药物等各个方面，构成了一整套合乎客观实际的医疗方法，灵活地指导着中医临床的实践。

Transliteration 1.1

Zhōng-yī yòng yīn yáng xué-shuō lái shuō-míng yī-xué shàng-de jī-běn wèn-tí, cóng-ér chéng-wéi zhōng-yī lǐ-lùn de sī-xiǎng tǐ-xì, tā guàn-chuàn zài zhōng-yī-xué zhōng de shēng-lǐ, bìng-lǐ, zhěn-duàn, zhì-liáo hé yào-wù děng gè-ge fāng-miàn, gòu-chéng le yī zhěng-tào hé-hū kè-guān shí-jì de yī-liáo fāng-fǎ, líng-huó de zhǐ-dǎo zhe zhōng-yī lín-chuáng de shí-jiàn.

Vocabulary 1.1

中	zhōng	Chinese
医	yī	medicine
中医	zhōng-yī	Chinese medicine
用	yòng	employ; use
阴阳	yīn yáng	yin and yang (the two principles and basic categories of all being)
学说	xué-shuō	theory; doctrine
来	lái	in order to
说明	shuō-míng	explain
医学	yī-xué	medicine
的	de	(particle defining the immediately preceding expression as a state of being)
上的	shàng-de	being present in ...; concerning
基本	jī-běn	basic
问题	wèn-tí	issue; question
从而	cóng-ér	hence; therefore
成为	chéng-wéi	constitute
理论	lǐ-lùn	theory
的	de	(particle defining a possessive)
思想	sī-xiǎng	thought; idea
体系	tǐ-xì	system
它	tā	it
贯串	guàn-chuàn	permeate; penetrate
在	zài	in; at
中	zhōng	in; amidst
在 ... 中的	zài ... zhōng de	being present in ...
中医学	zhōng-yī-xué	Chinese medicine
生理	shēng-lǐ	physiology
病理	bìng-lǐ	pathology
诊断	zhěn-duàn	diagnosis
治疗	zhì-liáo	treat; therapy

和	hé	and
药物	yào-wù	pharmaceutics; medical drugs
等	děng	(particle defining the end of an enumeration)
各个	gè-ge	each
方面	fāng-miàn	aspect
构成	gòu-chéng	constitute
了	le	(resultative particle highlighting a new situation)
一	yī	one
整套	zhěng-tào	complete system; set
合乎	hé-hū	conform
客观	kè-guān	objective
实际	shí-jì	reality
医疗	yī-liáo	treat; therapy
方法	fāng-fǎ	method
灵活	líng-huó	adaptable; flexible
地	de	(particle defining the immediately preceding expression as an adverb; roughly equivalent to the English "..ly")
指导	zhǐ-dǎo	guide
着	zhe	(particle defining the immediately preceding verb as a gerund; roughly equivalent to the English "..ing")
临床	lín-chuáng	clinical
实践	shí-jiàn	practice

Translation 1.1

Chinese medicine employs the yinyang doctrine to explain basic issues in the realm of medicine. Hence (the yinyang doctrine) constitutes the system of ideas of Chinese medical theory. It permeates all aspects of Chinese medicine, including physiology, pathology, diagnosis, therapy, and pharmaceutics. Hence it constitutes a complete therapeutic method that conforms to objective reality and provides adaptable guidance in the clinical practice of Chinese medicine.

Text 1.2

阴阳学说，是古人在观察自然现象中归纳出来，用以解释自然现象的一种思想方法。前人发现万物万象都有正反两种属性，这种属性是对立而又统一的，普遍存在于一切事物中，就创立了阴阳学说，用阴阳这个名词来代表一切事物中所存在着的对立统一的关系。如天为阳，地为阴；日为阳，月为阴；昼为阳，夜为阴；火为阳，水为阴等，并用相反相成，对立统一的道理去解释宇宙间一切事物的变化。

Transliteration 1.2

Yīn yáng xué-shuō, shì gǔ-rén zài guān-chá zì-rán xiàn-xiàng zhōng guī-nà chū-lái, yòng yǐ jiě-shì zì-rán xiàn-xiàng de yī zhǒng sī-xiǎng fāng-fǎ. Qián-rén fā-xiàn wàn-wù wàn-xiàng dōu yǒu zhèng-fǎn liǎng zhǒng shǔ-xìng, zhè zhǒng shǔ-xìng shì duì-lì ér yòu tǒng-yī de, pǔ-biàn cún-zài yú yī-qiè shì-wù zhōng, jiù chuàng-lì le yīn yáng xué-shuō, yòng yīn yáng zhè ge míng-cí lái dài-biǎo yī-qiè shì-wù zhōng suǒ cún-zài zhe de duì-lì tǒng-yī de guān-xi. Rú tiān wéi yáng, dì wéi yīn; rì wéi yáng, yuè wéi yīn; zhòu wéi yáng, yè wéi yīn; huǒ wéi yáng, shuǐ wéi yīn děng, bìng yòng xiāng-fǎn xiāng-chéng, duì-lì tǒng-yī de dào-lǐ qù jiě-shì yǔ-zhòu jiān yī-qiè shì-wù de biàn-huà.

Vocabulary 1.2

是	shì	be; is
古	gǔ	old; antiquity
人	rén	man
古人	gǔ-rén	people of antiquity; the ancients
观察	guān-chá	observe
自然	zì-rán	nature; natural
现象	xiàn-xiàng	phenomenon
归纳	guī-nà	draw inductive conclusions
出来	chū-lái	lit.: come out (particle indicating the outcome of a process indicated by the immediately preceding verb)
以	yǐ	in order to; for
解释	jiě-shì	explain
种	zhǒng	type; (measure word for abstract concepts)
前	qián	first; former
前人	qián-rén	people of former times
发现	fā-xiàn	find; discover
万	wàn	ten thousand

万物	wàn-wù	all things; myriad
万象	wàn-xiàng	all phenomena; myriad phenomena
都	dōu	all
有	yǒu	have; exist
正	zhèng	proper; regular; normal
反	fǎn	opposite
正反	zhèng-fǎn	norm and opposite
两	liǎng	two
属性	shǔ-xìng	attribute
这	zhè	this; these
对立	duì-lì	antagonistic
而	ér	and; and yet
又	yòu	still; again
统一	tǒng-yī	united; unity
普遍	pǔ-biàn	universal; ubiquitous; general
存在	cún-zài	be present; exist
于	yú	at; in
一切	yī-qiè	all; each
事物	shì-wù	thing; item
就	jiù	(particle indicating a subsequent process as an obvious consequence of a condition mentioned before)
创立	chuàng-lì	establish; found
了	le	(particle defining the immediately preceding verb as past tense)
个	ge	(general measure word)
名词	míng-cí	designation; name; term
代表	dài-biǎo	represent
所	suǒ	(relative pronoun)
关系	guān-xi	relationship
如	rú	for example; e.g.; be like
天	tiān	heaven

为	wéi	be; is
日	rì	sun
月	yuè	moon
昼	zhòu	daytime
夜	yè	night
火	huǒ	fire
水	shuǐ	water
并	bìng	simultaneous
相	xiāng	mutual
相反	xiāng-fǎn	be mutually opposite
成	chéng	constitute
相成	xiāng-chéng	be mutually complementary
道理	dào-lǐ	principle
去	qù	go; in order to
宇宙	yǔ-zhòu	universe
间	jiān	between; amidst; in
变化	biàn-huà	change

Translation 1.2

The yinyang doctrine is a way of thinking developed by the ancients through inductive conclusions from observing natural phenomena, and it is used to explain these natural phenomena. Our forefathers discovered that all things and all phenomena have the two attributes of norm and opposite, that these attributes are antagonistic though unified, and that (these attributes) exist ubiquitously in all things. (Hence the ancients) established the yinyang doctrine, and they made use of the two terms yin and yang to represent all relationships of antagonism and (simultaneous) unity that exist among all things. For instance, heaven is yang, the earth is yin; the sun is yang, the moon is yin; daytime is yang, the night is yin; fire is yang, water is yin. In addition, (the ancients) made use of the principles of (all things) being (both) opposite and complimentary to each other, (that is the principle) of antagonism and (simultaneous) unity, to interprete the changes that all things of the universe undergo.

在生理方面：中医认为人体的生理也能用阴阳学说来加以解释。一般的说，阳的性质属于动，阴的性质属于静；阳有保卫体表的能力，阴有保守内部精气的作用。故在生理上，以阳代表体表皮毛，肌肉，筋骨等，以阴代表体内脏腑；并以五脏主藏精气为阴，六腑主司消化传导为阳。又从位置上分：上焦为阳，下焦为阴；外侧为阳，内侧为阴。从物质和功能上分：血为阴，气为阳。每一处都存在着阴阳的属性，用以说明生理的特有的性质和特殊的功能。

Transliteration 1.3

Zài shēng-lǐ fāng-miàn: zhōng-yī rèn-wéi rén-tǐ de shēng-lǐ yě néng yòng yīn yáng xué-shuō lái jiā-yǐ jiě-shì. Yī-bān-de-shuō, yáng de xìng-zhì shǔ-yú dòng, yīn de xìng-zhì shǔ-yú jìng; yáng yǒu bǎo-wèi tǐ-biǎo de néng-lì, yīn yǒu bǎo-shǒu nèi-bù jīng-qì de zuò-yòng. Gù zài shēng-lǐ shàng, yǐ yáng dài-biǎo tǐ-biǎo pí máo, jī ròu, jīn gǔ děng, yǐ yīn dài-biǎo tǐ-nèi zàng-fǔ; bìng yǐ wǔ-zàng zhǔ cáng jīng-qì wéi yīn, liù-fǔ zhǔ-sī xiāo-huà chuán-dǎo wéi yáng. Yòu cóng wèi-zhì shàng fēn: shàng-jiāo wéi yáng, xià-jiāo wéi yīn; wài-cè wéi yáng, nèi-cè wéi yīn. Cóng wù-zhì hé gōng-néng shàng fēn: xuè wéi yīn, qì wéi yáng. Měi-yī chù dōu cún-zài zhe yīn yáng de shǔ-xìng, yòng yǐ shuō-míng shēng-lǐ de tè-yǒu de xìng-zhì hé tè-shū de gōng-néng.

Vocabulary 1.3

在 ... 方面	zài ... fāng-miàn	as for ...
认为	rèn-wéi	deem; think; consider; hold
人体	rén-tǐ	the human body
也	yě	too; also
能	néng	be able; can
用 ... 来	yòng ... lái	with
加以	jiā-yǐ	(an expression defining the immediately preceding statement as an object of the following verb; often intranslatable)
一般的说	yī-bān-de-shuō	generally speaking

性质	xìng-zhì	quality; nature
属于	shǔ-yú	be associated with; belong to
动	dòng	move; movement
静	jìng	rest; quietude
保卫	bǎo-wèi	safeguard; protect
表	biǎo	exterior; outer side
体表	tǐ-biǎo	the body's exterior
能力	néng-lì	ability
保守	bǎo-shǒu	protect; maintain
内部	nèi-bù	inner section
精气	jīng-qì	essential qi
作用	zuò-yòng	function; effect
在 ... 上	zài ... shàng	in ...; as for ...
故	gù	hence; therefore
上	shàng	on; in
以	yǐ	take; by means of
皮	pí	skin
毛	máo	hair
肌	jī	muscle
肉	ròu	flesh
筋	jīn	sinew
骨	gǔ	bone
内	nèi	inner; inside; interior
体内	tǐ-nèi	the body's interior
以 A 为 B	yǐ A wéi B	consider A as B
脏腑	zàng-fǔ	the inner organs
五	wǔ	five
五脏	wǔ-zàng	the five depots (i.e., lung, heart, spleen, liver, kidney)
主	zhǔ	master; be responsible for
藏	cáng	store
六	liù	six
六腑	liù-fǔ	the six palaces (i.e., gallbladder, bladder, stomach, small

		intestine, large intestine, triple burner)
主司	zhǔ-sī	be responsible for
消	xiāo	dissolve
化	huà	transform
消化	xiāo-huà	digest; digestion
传导	chuán-dǎo	transmit; transmission
从	cóng	from
位置	wèi-zhì	location
分	fēn	differentiate; order
上焦	shàng-jiāo	the upper burner
下	xià	below
下焦	xià-jiāo	the lower burner
侧	cè	side
外侧	wài-cè	outer side
内侧	nèi-cè	inner side
物质	wù-zhì	matter; substance
功能	gōng-néng	function
血	xuè	blood
气	qì	qi
每一	měi-yī	each; any
处	chù	locality
特有	tè-yǒu	characteristic; unique
特殊	tè-shū	specific; special

Translation 1.3

As for physiology, Chinese medicine holds that the physiology of the human body can also be explained with the yinyang doctrine. Generally speaking, the nature of yang is associated with movement, while the nature of yin is associated with rest. Yang has the ability of safeguarding the body's exterior; yin has the function of protecting the essential qi[1] of the interior section. Hence in physiology, yang represents the skin and the hair, the muscles and the flesh, as well as the sinews and the bones in the body's exterior, while yin represents the depots and palaces in the body's interior. In addition, (Chinese medicine) considers the five depots as yin because they master the storage of essential qi, and it considers the six palaces as yang because they are responsible for digestion and transmission. Furthermore, a distinction is made on the basis of locations: the upper burner is yang; the lower burner is yin.[2] Any outer side is yang; any inner side is yin. There are differentiations on the basis of substance and function: blood is yin; qi is yang. The yin or yang nature inherent in any locality is used to elucidate characteristic qualities and specific functions in physiology.

Notes

1 The concept of "qi" is explained in more detail in Lesson 5.

2 On the concept of the "Triple Burner" see Text 4.7.

Text 1.4

在病理方面：根据发病的部位和性质，区别表症属阳，里症属阴；热症属阳，寒症属阴。凡是机能衰弱，如少气，懒言，怕冷，疲倦，不耐劳动等多为阳的不足；物质的损失，如贫血，萎黄，遗精，消瘦等多为阴的不足。因而把一般症状分作四个类型，即阳虚，阴虚，阳盛，阴盛。概括地说，一切亢进的，兴奋的，有热性倾向的都归阳症，衰弱的，潜伏的，有寒性倾向的都归阴症。推而至于外科，阳症多是红肿发热，阴症多是白陷不发热。

Transliteration 1.4

Zài bìng-lǐ fāng-miàn: gēn-jù fā-bìng de bù-wèi hé xìng-zhì, qū-bié biǎo-zhèng shǔ yáng, lǐ-zhèng shǔ yīn; rè-zhèng shǔ yáng, hán-zhèng shǔ yīn. Fán-shì jī-néng shuāi-ruò, rú shǎo-qì, lǎn-yán, pà-lěng, pí-juàn, bù nài láo-dòng děng duō wéi yáng de bù-zú; wù-zhì de sǔn-shī, rú pín-xuè, wěi-huáng, yí-jīng, xiāo-shòu děng duō wéi yīn de bù-zú. Yīn-ér bǎ yī-bān zhèng-zhuàng fēn-zuò sì ge lèi-xíng, jí yáng-xū, yīn-xū, yáng-shèng, yīn-shèng. Gài-kuò-de-shuō, yī-qiè kàng-jìn de, xīng-fèn de, yǒu rè-xìng qīng-xiàng de dōu guī yáng-zhèng, shuāi-ruò de, qián-fú de, yǒu hán-xìng qīng-xiàng de dōu guī yīn-zhèng. Tuī-ér-zhì-yú wài-kē, yáng-zhèng duō shì hóng-zhǒng fā-rè, yīn-zhèng duō shì bái xiàn bù fā-rè.

Vocabulary 1.4

根据	gēn-jù	on the basis of; in accordance with; basis
发	fā	develop; appear
病	bìng	illness
发病	fā-bìng	breakout of an illness
部位	bù-wèi	location
区别	qū-bié	distinguish
症	zhèng	pathocondition
表症	biǎo-zhèng	pathoconditions affecting the body's exterior
属	shǔ	belong to

里症	lǐ-zhèng	pathoconditions affecting the body's interior
热症	rè-zhèng	pathoconditions of heat
寒	hán	cold
寒症	hán-zhèng	pathoconditions of cold
凡是	fán-shì	all; whenever
机能	jī-néng	function
衰弱	shuāi-ruò	weak
少	shǎo	few; little
气	qì	breath
少气	shǎo-qì	short of breath
懒言	lǎn-yán	laziness to talk
怕	pà	fear
冷	lěng	cold
怕冷	pà-lěng	aversion to cold
疲倦	pí-juàn	fatigue
不	bù	not
耐	nài	endure
劳动	láo-dòng	work; toil
多	duō	many; often
不足	bù-zú	insufficient
损失	sǔn-shī	lose
贫	pín	poor; lacking
贫血	pín-xuè	anemia
萎黄	wěi-huáng	sallow-yellow (complexion)
遗	yí	lose
精	jīng	essence; semen
遗精	yí-jīng	seminal emission
消瘦	xiāo-shòu	emaciation
因而	yīn-ér	hence
把	bǎ	(particle identifying the immediately following expression as an object of the subsequent verb)
一般	yī-bān	in general; generally

症状	zhèng-zhuàng	pathomanifestation
分作	fēn-zuò	categorize
四	sì	four
类型	lèi-xíng	type
即	jí	namely; that is
阳虚	yáng-xū	yang depletion
阴虚	yīn-xū	yin depletion
阳盛	yáng-shèng	yang abundance
阴盛	yīn-shèng	yin abundance
概括地说	gài-kuò-de-shuō	generally speaking; to put it briefly
亢进	kàng-jìn	hyperfunction
兴奋	xīng-fèn	exitement
热	rè	hot; heat
性	xìng	nature
热性	rè-xìng	hot nature
倾向	qīng-xiàng	tendency
归	guī	identify as
阳症	yáng-zhèng	yang pathocondition
潜伏	qián-fú	hidden; invisible
寒性	hán-xìng	cold nature
推而至于	tuī-ér-zhì-yú	as for ...
外	wài	outside; external
科	kē	scientific or medical speciality
外科	wài-kē	medical speciality concerned with external illnesses
红	hóng	red; reddening
肿	zhǒng	swell; swelling
发热	fā-rè	develop a fever; fever
阴症	yīn-zhèng	yin pathocondition
白	bái	white
陷	xiàn	sink in

Translation 1.4

As for pathology, on the basis of the location where illnesses develop, and (also on the basis of their) nature, (Chinese medicine) distinguishes between pathoconditions[1] affecting the exterior which belong to the yang, and pathoconditions affecting the interior which belong to the yin, pathoconditions of heat which belong to the yang, and pathoconditions of cold which belong to the yin. Whenever functions are weakened, as in case of shortness of breath, laziness to talk, aversion to cold, fatigue, and also inability to work, this is often an insufficiency of yang. Losses of substance, as in case of anemia, sallow-yellow (complexion), seminal emission, or emaciation, this is often an insufficiency of yin. Hence (Chinese medicine) categorizes the common pathomanifestations[2] into four types, namely yang depletion, yin depletion, yang abundance, and yin abundance. To put it briefly, all (cases) of a hyperfunction, of an excitement, and those having a tendency of a hot nature are identified as yang pathoconditions. All (cases) of weakness, of hidden (illnesses), and those having a tendency of a cold nature are identified as yin pathoconditions. In the (medical) speciality concerned with external (illnesses), yang pathoconditions often consist of reddening, swellings, and fever, while yin pathoconditions often appear as white or sunken (skin), and not as fever.

Notes

1 The term zhèng ("pathocondition") will be employed in the following texts with two meanings. First with the historical meaning of a real pathological condition noticeable for the patient as sign of an illness which itself remains unnoticeable to the patient. An example is an insufficient presence of yin accompanied by emaciation. The insufficiency of yin is the illness which itself cannot be perceived by the patient as such. The emaciation is the "pathocondition," which can be perceived by the patient very well as change in his subjective feeling of wellbeing. This historical meaning of the term zhèng is no longer strictly applied in contemporary Chinese literature on traditional Chinese medicine. Nowadays the term zhèng often stands for the pathology, i.e., the illness, itself.

2 The term zhèng-zhuàng is not documented in pre-modern texts of Chinese medicine; it was introduced in the context of Western medicine and is commonly translated as "symptom." In the present text it is used synonymously with zhèng, "pathocondition." Because the concept of zhèng in Chinese medicine does not entirely correspond to that of "symptom" in Western medicine, the use of the latter term is avoided here.

Text 1.5

在诊断上：如以脉诊来说，分有六个纲要，即在至数上分迟和数，体状上分浮和沉，动态上分滑和涩。数，浮，滑属于阳，迟，沉，涩属于阴；阴脉多见于阴症，阳脉多见于阳症。以舌诊来说，舌质的变化属于血液的病变，色见红，绛，乃是血热属阳，色淡或青，乃是血虚或血寒属阴；舌苔的变化多系肠胃的病变，燥的黄的属阳，潮的白的属阴。

Transliteration 1.5

Zài zhěn-duàn shàng: rú yǐ mài-zhěn lái shuō, fēn-yǒu liù ge gāng-yào, jí zài zhì-shù shàng fēn chí hé shuò, tǐ-zhuàng shàng fēn fú hé chén, dòng-tài shàng fēn huá hé sè. Shuò, fú, huá shǔ-yú yáng, chí, chén, sè shǔ-yú yīn;

yīn-mài duō jiàn yú yīn-zhèng, yáng-mài duō jiàn yú yáng-zhèng. Yǐ shé-zhěn lái shuō, shé-zhì de biàn-huà shǔ-yú xuè-yè de bìng-biàn, sè jiàn hóng, jiàng, nǎi-shì xuè-rè shǔ yáng, sè dàn huò qīng, nǎi-shì xuè-xū huò xuè-hán shǔ yīn; shé-tāi de biàn-huà duō xì cháng wèi de bìng-biàn, zào de huáng de shǔ yáng, cháo de bái de shǔ yīn.

Vocabulary 1.5

脉诊	mài-zhěn	pulse diagnosis
以 ... 来说	yǐ ... lái shuō	as far as ... is concerned
分有	fēn-yǒu	distinguish
纲要	gāng-yào	fundamental categories
至	zhì	arrive; reach
数	shù	number
至数	zhì-shù	pulse frequency (arrival of pulses)
迟	chí	retarded; slow
数	shuò	frequent; accelerated
体状	tǐ-zhuàng	physical appearance
浮	fú	at the surface
沉	chén	deep
动态	dòng-tài	nature of movement
滑	huá	smooth
涩	sè	rough
阴脉	yīn-mài	yin pulse
见	jiàn	appear
阳脉	yáng-mài	yang pulse
舌	shé	tongue
诊	zhěn	examine; diagnose
舌诊	shé-zhěn	tongue diagnosis
舌质	shé-zhì	tongue substance
液	yè	liquid
血液	xuè-yè	blood
变	biàn	change

病变	bìng-biàn	pathological change
色	sè	color
绛	jiàng	crimson
乃是	nǎi-shì	that is; then it is ...
血热	xuè-rè	blood heat
淡	dàn	pale
或	huò	or
青	qīng	virid
血虚	xuè-xū	blood depletion
血寒	xuè-hán	blood cold
舌苔	shé-tāi	tongue coating
系	xì	belong to
肠	cháng	intestine
胃	wèi	stomach
燥	zào	parched
黄	huáng	yellow
潮	cháo	moist

Translation 1.5

In diagnosis, as far as pulse diagnosis is concerned, (Chinese medicine) distinguishes between six fundamental categories. That is, with regard to the pulse frequency it distinguishes between retarded and frequent, with regard to physical appearance it distinguishes between at the surface and deep, and with regard to nature of movement it distinguishes between smooth and rough. Frequent (pulses, pulses) at the surface, and smooth (pulses) belong to the yang; retarded (pulses), deep (pulses), and rough (pulses) belong to the yin. Yin pulses often appear with yin pathoconditions; yang pulses often appear together with yang pathoconditions. As far as tongue diagnosis is concerned, changes in the tongue substance are associated with pathological changes of the blood. If a red or crimson color appears, these are (signs of) blood heat; they belong to the yang. If the color is pale or virid, then this is a blood depletion or blood cold, and (such states) belong to the yin. Changes of the tongue coating are often tied to pathological changes of the intestines and/or the stomach. A parched or yellow (coating) belongs to the yang; a moist or white (coating) belongs to the yin.

Text 1.6

在治疗上：表症用汗法，里症用下法，寒症用温法，热症用凉法，都含有阴阳的意义。主要是阳胜则阴病，阴胜则阳病；阳胜则热，阴胜则寒，重寒能现热象，重热能现寒象。

Transliteration 1.6

Zài zhì-liáo shàng: biǎo-zhèng yòng hàn-fǎ, lǐ-zhèng yòng xià-fǎ, hán-zhèng yòng wēn-fǎ, rè-zhèng yòng liáng-fǎ, dōu hán-yǒu yīn yáng de yì-yì. Zhǔ-yào shì yáng-shèng zé yīn-bìng, yīn-shèng zé yáng bìng; yáng-shèng zé rè, yīn-shèng zé hán, chóng-hán néng xiàn rè-xiàng, chóng-rè néng xiàn hán-xiàng.

Vocabulary 1.6

汗	hàn	sweat; perspiration
法	fǎ	(therapeutic) pattern
汗法	hàn-fǎ	(therapeutic) pattern inducing perspiration
下	xià	down; downwards; descend
下法	xià-fǎ	(therapeutic) pattern causing a downward movement; purging

温	wēn	warm
温法	wēn-fǎ	(therapeutic) pattern causing a warming
凉	liáng	cool
凉法	liáng-fǎ	cooling (therapy) pattern
含有	hán-yǒu	include
意义	yì-yì	meaning; significance
主要	zhǔ-yào	basically; in principle
胜	shèng	dominate
阳胜	yáng-shèng	yang domination
则	zé	then
阴病	yīn-bìng	yin illness
阴胜	yīn-shèng	yin domination
阳病	yáng-bìng	yang illness
重	chóng	doubled
重寒	chóng-hán	doubled cold
现	xiàn	bring forth; cause to appear
热象	rè-xiàng	heat signs
重热	chóng-rè	doubled heat
寒象	hán-xiàng	cold signs

Translation 1.6

In therapy, (Chinese medicine) applies patterns inducing perspiration in cases of pathoconditions affecting the exterior, and it applies patterns causing a downward purging in cases of pathoconditions affecting the interior. In cases of pathoconditions of cold, it employs a warming pattern; in cases of pathoconditions of heat, it employs a cooling pattern. All (these patterns) have a significance in terms of the yinyang (doctrine). In principle, when yang dominates, then the yin has an illness; when the yin dominates, then the yang has an illness: When the yang dominates, then heat (develops); when the yin dominates, then cold (develops). Doubled cold may cause heat signs to appear; doubled heat may cause cold signs to appear.

Text 1.7

在用药方面：中药的药性主要是分别气味。一般以气为阳，味为阴。气又分四种，寒，凉属阴，温，热属阳；味分五种，辛，甘属阳，酸，苦，咸属阴。故附子，肉桂，干姜等具有辛热性的称做阳药，能升能散；黄连，银花，龙胆草等具有苦寒性的称做阴药，能降能泻。此外，有芳香健胃作用的如砂仁，豆蔻等，也叫做阳药，有滋养肝肾作用的如首乌，地黄等，也叫做阴药。

Transliteration 1.7

Zài yòng-yào fāng-miàn: zhōng-yào de yào-xìng zhǔ-yào shì fēn-bié qì wèi. Yī-bān yǐ qì wéi yáng, wèi wéi yīn. Qì yòu fēn sì zhǒng, hán, liàng shǔ yīn, wēn, rè shǔ yáng; wèi fēn wǔ zhǒng, xīn, gān shǔ yáng, suān, kǔ, xián shǔ yīn. Gù fù-zǐ, ròu-guì, gān-jiāng děng jù-yǒu xīn rè-xìng de chēng-zuò yáng-yào, néng shēng néng sàn; huáng-lián, yín-huā, lóng-dǎn-cǎo děng jù-yǒu kǔ hán-xìng de chēng-zuò yīn-yào, néng jiàng néng xiè. Cǐ-wài, yǒu fāng-xiāng jiàn wèi zuò-yòng de rú shā-rén, dòu-kòu děng, yě jiào-zuò yáng-yào, yǒu zī-yǎng gān shèn zuò-yòng de rú shǒu-wū, dì-huáng děng, yě jiào-zuò yīn-yào.

Vocabulary 1.7

药	yào	drug
用药	yòng-yào	drug use
中药	zhōng-yào	traditional Chinese drug
药性	yào-xìng	drug quality
分别	fēn-bié	differentiate
气	qì	qi (drug quality)
味	wèi	flavor (drug quality)
辛	xīn	acrid
甘	gān	sweet
酸	suān	sour
苦	kǔ	bitter
咸	xián	salty
附子	fù-zǐ	(drug name) Aconitum carmichaeli Debx.
肉桂	ròu-guì	(drug name) Cinnamomum cassia Presl.
干姜	gān-jiāng	(drug name) dried ginger
具有	jù-yǒu	possess; have
称做 (作)	chēng-zuò	be called; call
阴药	yīn-yào	yin drug

升	shēng	ascend
散	sàn	disperse
黄连	huáng-lián	(drug name) Coptis chinensis Franch.
银花	yín-huā	(drug name) Lonicera japonica Thunb. L.
龙胆草	lóng-dǎn-cǎo	(drug name) Gentiana scabra Bge.
降	jiàng	sink
泻	xiè	drain
此外	cǐ-wài	furthermore
芳香	fāng-xiāng	fragrant; aromatic
健	jiàn	strengthen
砂仁	shā-rén	(drug name) Amomum xanthioides Wall.
豆蔻	dòu-kòu	(drug name) Amomum cardamomum L.
叫做	jiào-zuò	be called; call
阳药	yáng-yào	yang drug
滋养	zī-yǎng	nourish
肝	gān	liver
肾	shèn	kidneys
首乌	shǒu-wū	(drug name) Polygonum multiflorum Thunb.
地黄	dì-huáng	(drug name) Rhemannia glutinosa (Gaertn.) Libosch.

Translation 1.7

As for the use of drugs, there is a basic differentiation in the qualities of drugs of Chinese pharmaceutics between qi[1] and flavor. In general, qi is classified as yang, flavor as yin. Among the qi, again, four types are distinguished: cold and cool are associated with yin; warm and hot are associated with yang. Among the flavors five types are distinguished: acrid and sweet are associated with the yang; sour, bitter, and salty are associated with the yin. Hence (such drugs as) fuzi, rougui, and ganjiang which possess acrid and hot qualities are called yang drugs; they are able to ascend (in the organism) and to disperse. Huanglian, yinhua, and longdancao which possess bitter and cold qualities are called yin drugs. They are able to sink (in the organism) and to drain. Furthermore, (substances) like sharen and doukou who are fragrant and which have the function of strengthening the stomach are also called yang drugs, while (substances) like shouwu and dihuang which have the function of nourishing the liver and the kidneys are also called yin drugs.

Note

1 On the meaning of qi as drug quality, see Text 16.5

Text 1.8

阴阳既是事物对立统一的概括性代名词，故不论物质的，机能的，部位的对立，都可以包括。不过应该明确中医广泛地把阴阳应用于各个方面，都是实有所指的，因此要彻底理解中医运用阴阳的道理，必须通过临症，只有通过临症才能明白阴阳所起的实际作用。例如热是属于阳，但热有表里，虚实的不同，故伤风感冒引起的发热，当用发汗法，叫做疏散解表；化脓性肿疡引起的发热，当用内消法，叫做消散清解；肝火引起的发热，当用清降法，叫做平肝清热。所以，热属于阳这是一般情况，而热的属于表，属于里，属于虚，属于实则是机动的。

Transliteration 1.8

Yīn yáng jì shì shì-wù duì-lì tǒng-yī de gài-kuò-xìng dài-míng-cí, gù bù-lùn wù-zhì de, jī-néng de, bù-wèi de duì-lì, dōu kě-yǐ bāo-kuò. Bù-guò yīng-gāi míng-què zhōng-yī guǎng-fàn de bǎ yīn yáng yīng yòng yú gè-ge fāng-miàn, dōu-shì shí yǒu suǒ zhǐ de, yīn-cǐ yào chè-dǐ lǐ-jiě zhōng-yī yùn-yòng yīn yáng de dào-lǐ, bì-xū tōng-guò lín-zhèng, zhǐ-yǒu tōng-guò lín-zhèng cái néng míng-bái yīn yáng suǒ qǐ de shí-jì zuò-yòng. Lì-rú rè shì shǔ-yú yáng, dàn rè yǒu biǎo lǐ, xū shí de bù-tóng, gù shāng-fēng gǎn-mào yǐn-qǐ de fā-rè, dāng yòng fā-hàn-fǎ, jiào-zuò shū-sàn jiě-biǎo; huà-nóng-xìng zhǒng-yáng yǐn-qǐ de fā-rè, dāng yòng nèi-xiāo-fǎ, jiào-zuò xiāo-sàn qīng-jiě; gān-huǒ yǐn-qǐ de fā-rè, dāng yòng qīng-jiàng-fǎ, jiào-zuò píng-gān qīng-rè. Suǒ-yǐ, rè shǔ-yú yáng zhè shì yī-bān qíng-kuàng, ér rè de shǔ-yú biǎo, shǔ-yú lǐ, shǔ-yú xū, shǔ-yú shí zé shì jī-dòng de.

Vocabulary 1.8

既	jì	since
概括性	gài-kuò-xìng	general
代名词	dài-míng-cí	synonym
不论	bù-lùn	regardless
可以	kě-yǐ	can; be able
包括	bāo-kuò	include

不过	bù-guò	however
应该	yīng-gāi	should, must
明确	míng-què	make clear; emphasize
广泛	guǎng-fàn	extensive; comprehensive
应用	yìng-yòng	apply
都是	dōu-shì	always; all; in each case
实有	shí-yǒu	fact
指	zhǐ	refer to
因此	yīn-cǐ	hence
彻底	chè-dǐ	carefully
理解	lǐ-jiě	understand
运用	yùn-yòng	apply
必须	bì-xū	must
例如	lì-rú	for example
通过	tōng-guò	pass through
临症	lín-zhèng	clinical (experience)
只有	zhǐ-yǒu	only if
才	cái	then
明白	míng-bái	understand
起	qǐ	bring forth; set off
但	dàn	but
里	lǐ	inner
虚	xū	depletion
实	shí	repletion
不同	bù-tóng	different
伤	shāng	harm
风	fēng	wind
伤风	shāng-fēng	harm caused by wind
感冒	gǎn-mào	common cold
引起	yǐn-qǐ	cause; set off
实	shí	fact; reality
当	dāng	should; must
发汗法	fā-hàn-fǎ	(therapeutic) pattern inducing perspiration
疏散	shū-sàn	disperse; dispersion

解	jiě	open; loosen
解表	jiě-biǎo	open the exterior
化	huà	transform
脓	nóng	pus
化脓性	huà-nóng-xìng	suppurating
内消法	nèi-xiāo-fǎ	(therapeutic) pattern of internal elimination
消散	xiāo-sàn	elimination through dispersion
清解	qīng-jiě	cooling through opening
肝火	gān-huǒ	liver fire
清降法	qīng-jiàng-fǎ	(therapeutic) pattern for cooling and subduing (heat)
要	yào	wish
应	yīng	should, must
平	píng	even; level; calm
平肝	píng-gān	calm the liver
清	qīng	cool
清热	qīng-rè	cool the heat
所以	suǒ-yǐ	hence
情况	qíng-kuàng	condition
肿疡	zhǒng-yáng	lesion
机动	jī-dòng	adaptation; flexible; expedient

Translation 1.8

Since yin and yang are general synonyms for the antagonism with (simultaneous) unity among (all) things, they can include all antagonisms, regardless of whether these are those of matter, of function, or of position. However, it should be made clear that Chinese medicine in its extensive application of the yinyang (doctrine) to all realms, always refers to facts. Hence if (someone) wishes to thoroughly understand the principles of the application of the yinyang (doctrine) by Chinese medicine, he/she must pass through clinical (experience). Only through clinical (experience) is it possible to understand the practical applications emerging from the yinyang (doctrine). For example, heat is associated with yang. But there are differences of exterior and interior heat, of depletion and repletion heat. Hence in case of fever set off by harm caused by wind or common cold, a (therapeutic) pattern causing perspiration called "dispersing (heat) by opening the exterior" must be applied. In case of fever set off by suppurating lesions, a pattern of internal elimination called "elimination and dispersion, cooling and opening" must be applied. In case of fever set off by fire in the liver, a pattern to cool and subdue (the fire) called "to calm the liver, and to cool the heat" must be applied. That is to say, the association of heat and yang refers to a general condition, while the association of heat with the exterior or with the interior, with depletion or with repletion is a flexible adaptation (of the yinyang doctrine to specific situations).

Text 2.1

五行，即木，火，土，金，水。这五者的关系，主要有两个方面，即"相生"与"相克"。相生，就是相互资生和助长的关系。五行中的相生关系是这样的：木生火，火生土，土生金，金生水，水生木。从五行相生的关系中，可以看出，任何一行都有生我和我生两个方面，如以木为例，生我者为水，我生者为火，故借母子关系来说，水为木之母，火为木之子。其它四行以此类推。

Transliteration 2.1

Wǔ-xíng, jí mù, huǒ, tǔ, jīn, shuǐ. Zhè wǔ zhě de guān-xi, zhǔ-yào yǒu liǎng ge fāng-miàn, jí "xiāng-shēng" yǔ "xiāng-kè." Xiāng-shēng, jiù-shì xiāng-hù zī-shēng hé zhù-zhǎng de guān-xi. Wǔ-xíng zhōng de xiāng-shēng guān-xi shì zhè-yàng de: mù shēng huǒ, huǒ shēng tǔ, tǔ shēng jīn, jīn shēng shuǐ, shuǐ shēng mù. Cóng wǔ-xíng xiāng-shēng de guān-xi zhōng, kě-yǐ kàn-chū, rèn-hé yī xíng dōu yǒu shēng wǒ hé wǒ shēng liǎng ge fāng-miàn, rú yǐ mù wéi lì, shēng wǒ zhě wéi shuǐ, wǒ shēng zhě wéi huǒ, gù jiè mǔ zǐ guān-xi lái shuō, shuǐ wéi mù zhī mǔ, huǒ wéi mù zhī zǐ. Qí-tā sì xíng yǐ cǐ lèi-tuī.

Vocabulary 2.1

行	xíng	phase
五行	wǔ-xíng	the five phases
木	mù	wood
土	tǔ	soil
金	jīn	metal
者	zhě	(particle defining the immediately preceding verb or number as a noun referring to an item or to a person; here: wu zhe "the five;" zhe wu zhe "these five")
生	shēng	create; engender
相生	xiāng-shēng	mutual engendering
与	yǔ	and; with
克	kè	restrain
相克	xiāng-kè	mutual restraint
就是	jiù-shì	that is
相互	xiāng-hù	mutual
资生	zī-shēng	create
助长	zhù-zhǎng	support

这样	zhè-yàng	such
从 ... 中	cóng ... zhōng	from ...
看出	kàn-chū	recognize
任何一 ... 都	rèn-hé yī ... dōu	everybody; each
我	wǒ	I
例	lì	example
以 ... 为例	yǐ ... wéi lì	take ... as an example
借	jiè	make use of; borrow
借 ... 来说	jiè ... lái shuō	state in terms of ...
母	mǔ	mother
子	zǐ	son
之	zhī	(particle identifying the immediately preceding expression as a possessive)
其它	qí-tā	others
此	cǐ	this
类推	lèi-tuī	deduce analogously

Translation 2.1

The five phases are wood, fire, soil, metal, and water. The relationships among these five (phases) are marked by two basic aspects, namely (those of) "mutual engendering" and "mutual restraint." "Mutual engendering" is a relationship of mutual creation and support. The relationships of mutual engendering among the five phases are as follows: wood generates fire, fire generates soil, soil generates metal, metal generates water, water generates wood. From the relationships of mutual engendering among the five phases it is obvious that each single phase has two aspects, i.e., (some other phase) generates this (phase), and this (phase) generates (another phase). To take (the phase of) wood as an example, that (phase) which generates it is water, and that which it generates is fire. Hence speaking in terms of the mother-son relationship, water is the mother of wood, and fire is the son of wood. The (relationships among the) remaining four phases can be deduced analogously from this (example).

Text 2.2

相克，就是相互约制和克服的关系。五行中的相克关系是：金克木，木克土，土克水，水克火，火克金。在这五行相克的关系中，也可看出任何一行都有克我和我克两个方面，再以木为例，克我者为金，我克者为土，也就是金为木所"不胜"者，土为木所"胜"者。

Transliteration 2.2

Xiāng-kè, jiù-shì xiāng-hù yuē-zhì hé kè-fú de guān-xi. Wǔ-xíng zhōng de xiāng-kè guān-xi shì: jīn kè mù, mù kè tǔ, tǔ kè shuǐ, shuǐ kè huǒ, huǒ kè jīn. Zài zhè wǔ-xíng xiāng-kè de guān-xi zhōng, yě kě kàn-chū rèn-hé yī xíng dōu yǒu kè wǒ hé wǒ kè liǎng ge fāng-miàn, zài yǐ mù wéi lì, kè wǒ zhě wéi jīn, wǒ kè zhě wéi tǔ, yě-jiù-shì jīn wéi mù suǒ “bù-shèng” zhě, tǔ wéi mù suǒ “shèng” zhě.

Vocabulary 2.2

约制	yuē-zhì	restrict
克服	kè-fú	overcome
可	kě	can; be able
再	zài	again
也就是	yě-jiù-shì	in other words
A为B所	A wéi B suǒ ...	passive construction: A is ... by B

Translation 2.2

"Mutual restraint" is a relationship (where the five phases) restrict and overcome each other. The relationships of mutual restraint among the five phases are (the following): metal restrains wood, wood restrains soil, soil restrains water, water restrains fire, fire restrains metal. From these relationships of mutual restraint among the five phases it is obvious again that each phase has two aspects, i.e., (some other phase) restrains this (phase), and this (phase) restrains (another phase). To take wood as an example again, that which restrains this (phase) is metal, and that which it restrains is soil. That is, metal is that (phase) which wood "does not win against," while soil is that (phase) which wood "wins against."

Text 2.3

上述五行相生和相克两个方面，它们之间的关系，不是并行不悖，而是相互为用的，也就是生克之间有密切的联系，即生中有克，克中有生。这种相互为用的关系，称做"制化"关系，如：木克土，土生金，金克木。制化关系，是维持平衡的必要条件，否则有生无克，必使盛者更盛；有克无生，必使弱者更弱。

Transliteration 2.3

Shàng-shù wǔ-xíng xiāng-shēng hé xiāng-kè liǎng ge fāng-miàn, tā-men zhī-jiān de guān-xi, bù shì bìng-xíng-bù-bèi, ér shì xiāng-hù wéi yòng de, yě-jiù-shì shēng kè zhī-jiān yǒu mì-qiè de lián-xì, jí shēng zhōng yǒu kè, kè zhōng yǒu shēng. Zhè zhǒng xiāng-hù wéi yòng de guān-xi, chēng-zuò "zhì-huà" guān-xi, rú: mù kè tǔ, tǔ shēng jīn, jīn kè mù. Zhì-huà guān-xi, shì wéi-chí píng-héng de bì-yào tiáo-jiàn, fǒu-zé yǒu shēng wú kè, bì shǐ shèng zhě gèng shèng; yǒu kè wú shēng, bì shǐ ruò zhě gèng ruò.

Vocabulary 2.3

上述	shàng-shù	mentioned above
它们	tā-men	they
之间	zhī-jiān	among; between
并行不悖	bìng-xíng-bù-bèi	move in parallel without contact; coexist without affecting each other
密切	mì-qiè	close
联系	lián-xì	relationship
制化	zhì-huà	construction and counterreaction
维持	wéi-chí	maintain
平衡	píng-héng	balance
必要	bì-yào	necessary; essential
条件	tiáo-jiàn	condition; precondition
否则	fǒu-zé	if not then; otherwise
无	wú	have not; do not exist
必	bì	must; inevitably
使	shǐ	cause
盛	shèng	abundant
更	gèng	even more; further
弱	ruò	weak

Translation 2.3

The relationships among the two aspects of mutual engendering and mutual restraint of the five phases mentioned above are not such that (these two aspects merely) coexist without affecting each other; on the contrary, they are of use to each other. In other words, close relationships exist between engendering and restraint. That is, within engendering there is restraint, and within restraint there is engendering. These relationships of mutual use are called "construction and counterraction." For example, wood restrains soil, soil generates metal, metal restrains wood. The relationship of construction and counterreaction is an essential condition for maintaining a balance (among the phases). If it did not exist then there would be engendering without restraint, which would inevitably cause the abdundant to become even more abundant, or there would be restraint without engendering, which would inevitably cause the weak to become even weaker.

Text 2.4

在生克中还有一种反常现象，即我克者有时反来克我，克我者也有时反为我克。比如，水本克火，在某种情况下，火亦能反过来克水，这就称做"相侮"。凡是相生，相克，相侮均有一个条件，就是本身之气充实则相生，否则不能生；本身之气有余则能克所胜和侮所不胜，不及则不但不能克所胜而反为所不胜乘侮。

Transliteration 2.4

Zài shēng kè zhōng hái-yǒu yī zhǒng fǎn-cháng xiàn-xiàng, jí wǒ kè zhě yǒu-shí fǎn-lái kè wǒ, kè wǒ zhě yě yǒu-shí fǎn wéi wǒ kè. Bǐ-rú, shuǐ běn kè huǒ, zài mǒu-zhǒng qíng-kuàng xià, huǒ yì néng fǎn-guò-lái kè shuǐ, zhè jiù chēng-zuò "xiāng-wǔ."

Fán-shì xiāng-shēng, xiāng-kè, xiāng-wǔ jūn yǒu yī ge tiáo-jiàn, jiù-shì běn-shēn zhī qì chōng-shí zé xiāng-shēng, fǒu-zé bù néng shēng; běn-shēn zhī qì yǒu-yú zé néng kè suǒ shèng hé wǔ suǒ bù-shèng, bù-jí zé bù-dàn bù néng kè suǒ shèng ér fǎn wéi suǒ bù-shèng chéng wǔ.

Vocabulary 2.4

在 ... 中	zài ... zhōng	within ...
还	hái	still; in addition
还有	hái-yǒu	there is yet another ...
反常	fǎn-cháng	unusual
时	shí	time
有时	yǒu-shí	sometimes; occasionally
来	lái	come
反来	fǎn-lái	conversely; on the contrary
比如	bǐ-rú	for example
本	běn	origin; originally
在 ... 下	zài ... xià	under ...
某种	mǒu-zhǒng	certain
亦	yì	also
反过来	fǎn-guò-lái	conversely
侮	wǔ	rebel; hate; humiliate
相侮	xiāng-wǔ	mutual rebellion
均	jūn	all
身	shēn	body
本身	běn-shēn	itself
充实	chōng-shí	abundant
余	yú	surplus
有余	yǒu-yú	be present in surplus
不胜	bù-shèng	not to win
及	jí	reach
不及	bù-jí	insufficient
不但 ... 而	bù-dàn ... ér	not only ..., but ...

乘	chéng	seize; exploit (a weakness); take advantage

Translation 2.4

Within (these relationships of mutual) engendering and restraint, there is yet another unusual phenomenon, that is, (a phase) which (phase) A restrains, contrary (to what is normal), sometimes restrains (phase) A, and that (phase) which restrains (phase) A is also sometimes restrained by (phase) A. For example, in principle water restrains fire. Under certain conditions, fire – conversely – can restrain water; this (is a relationship) called "mutual humiliation." All these (relationships of) mutual engendering, mutual restraint, and mutual humiliation depend on a (specific) condition. That is, if the qi of (a specific phase) itself is abundant, then mutual engendering occurs. If this is not the case, then it cannot generate (another phase). If the qi of a (specific phase) itself is present in surplus, then it is able to restrain that which it wins against, and to humiliate that which it (usually) does not win against. If (the qi) is insufficient, then it will not only be unable to restrain that which it (usually) wins against, on the contrary it will be seized and humiliated by that (phase) which it (usually) does not win against.

Text 2.5

五行在中医学上的运用，主要是按五行的属性，将自然界和人体组织在一定的情况下归纳起来，同时以生克的关系说明脏腑之间的相互关系。就自然界来说，如方位的东，南，中，西，北，季节的春，夏，长夏，秋，冬，气候的风，暑，湿，燥，寒，生化过程的生，长，化，收，藏，以及五色的青，赤，黄，白，黑，五味的酸，苦，甘，辛，咸，均可依木，火，土，金，水的次序来从属。

Transliteration 2.5

Wǔ-xíng zài zhōng-yī-xué shàng-de yùn-yòng, zhǔ-yào shì àn wǔ-xíng de shǔ-xìng, jiāng zì-rán-jiè hé rén-tǐ-zǔ-zhī zài yī-dìng de qíng-kuàng xià guī-nà qǐ-lái, tóng-shí yǐ shēng kè de guān-xi shuō-míng zàng-fǔ zhī-jiān de xiāng-hù guān-xi. Jiù zì-rán-jiè lái shuō, rú fāng-wèi de dōng, nán, zhōng, xī, běi, jì-jié de chūn, xià, cháng-xià, qiū, dōng, qì-hòu de fēng, shǔ, shī, zào, hán, shēng-huà guò-chéng de shēng, zhǎng, huà, shōu, cáng, yǐ-jí wǔ-sè de qīng, chì, huáng, bái, hēi, wǔ-wèi de suān, kǔ, gān, xīn, xián, jūn kě yī mù, huǒ, tǔ, jīn, shuǐ de cì-xù lái cóng-shǔ.

Vocabulary 2.5

按	àn	in accordance with; according to
将	jiāng	(particle identifying the following expression as an object of the verb following that expression)
就 ... 来说	jiù ... lái shuō	take ... as an example
自然界	zì-rán-jiè	the natural world; nature
组织	zǔ-zhī	structure; tissue; organization
人体组织	rén-tǐ-zǔ-zhī	the human organism
一定	yī-dìng	definite; specific
起来	qǐ-lái	(particle emphasizing a moving towards above or an initial movement indicated by the immediately preceding verb)
同	tóng	identical; similar
同时	tóng-shí	at the same time
方位	fāng-wèi	position; cardinal point
东	dōng	east
南	nán	south
西	xī	west
北	běi	north
季节	jì-jié	season

春	chūn	spring
夏	xià	summer
长夏	cháng-xià	late summer
秋	qiū	autumn
冬	dōng	winter
气候	qì-hòu	climate
暑	shǔ	summerheat
湿	shī	dampness
生化	shēng-huà	lifecycle
过程	guò-chéng	process
长	zhǎng	grow; growth
收	shōu	shrink
以及	yǐ-jí	as well as; up to
赤	chì	red
黑	hēi	black
依	yī	depend on
依 ... 来	yī ... lái	in accordance with
次序	cì-xù	sequence
从属	cóng-shǔ	categorize

Translation 2.5

In principle, the application of the five phases (doctrine) in Chinese medicine is to conceptualize the natural world and the human organism under specific conditions in accordance with the characteristics of the five phases. At the same time, the relationships of engendering and restraint are used to explain the mutual relationships among the organs. To take the natural world as an example, east, south, center, west, and north (as dimensions) of the cardinal points, spring, summer, late summer, autumn, and winter (as dimensions) of the seasons, wind, summerheat, dampness, dryness, and cold (as dimensions) of the climate, birth, growth, transformation, shrinking, and passing away (as dimensions) of the lifecycle, as well as the five colors virid, red, yellow, white, and black, and the five flavors sour, bitter, sweet, acrid, and salty, they all can be categorized in accordance with the sequence wood, fire, soil, metal, and water (of the five phases).

Text 2.6

在人体方面，以肝，心，脾，肺，肾为中心，联系到目，舌，口，鼻，耳的七窍，筋，脉，肉，皮毛，骨的五体和怒，喜，思，忧，恐的五志等等。明白了这一归类方法后，当接触到属于某一行性质的事物时，便可从直接或间接的关系把它们结合起来加以分析，以便理解这一事物的性质。

Transliteration 2.6

Zài rén-tǐ fāng-miàn, yǐ gān, xīn, pí, fèi, shèn wéi zhōng-xīn, lián-xì dào mù, shé, kǒu, bí, ěr de qī-qiào, jīn, mài, ròu, pí máo, gǔ de wǔ-tǐ hé nù, xǐ, sī, yōu, kǒng de wǔ-zhì děng-děng. Míng-bái le zhè-yī guī-lèi fāng-fǎ hòu, dāng jiē-chù dào shǔ-yú mǒu-yī xíng xìng-zhì de shì-wù shí, biàn kě cóng zhí-jiē huò jiàn-jiē de guān-xi bǎ tā-men jié-hé qǐ-lái jiā-yǐ fēn-xī, yǐ-biàn lǐ-jiě zhè-yī shì-wù de xìng-zhì.

Vocabulary 2.6

心	xīn	heart
脾	pí	spleen
肺	fèi	lung
到	dào	to; with
目	mù	eye
口	kǒu	mouth
鼻	bí	nose
耳	ěr	ear
七窍	qī-qiào	the seven orifices
脉	mài	vessel
五体	wǔ-tǐ	the five (physical components constituting the) body
怒	nù	anger
喜	xǐ	joy
思	sī	thought
忧	yōu	anxiety
恐	kǒng	fear
五志	wǔ-zhì	the five minds
等等	děng-děng	and so on
这一	zhè-yī	this
归类	guī-lèi	categorize; classify
后	hòu	after
当 ... 时	dāng ... shí	at the time when ...
接触	jiē-chù	encounter
某一	mǒu-yī	a specific
便	biàn	(particle indicating that the fact referred to next results from a fact mentioned immediately before)
直接	zhí-jiē	direct
间接	jiàn-jiē	indirect
结合	jié-hé	link; connect
分析	fēn-xī	analyze

以便	yǐ-biàn	in order to

Translation 2.6

The human body is centered around liver, heart, spleen, lung, and kidneys, which are linked to the eyes, the tongue, the mouth, the nose, and the ears as the seven orifices, to the muscles, the vessels, the flesh, the skin, and the hair, as well as the bones as the five (physical components constituting the) body, to anger, joy, thought, anxiety, and fear as the five minds, and so on. Once this method of classification is understood, it will be possible, upon encountering an item that is related to the nature of a certain phase, to link them (i.e., item and phase) through direct or indirect relationships and, moreover, to carry out analyses to understand the nature of this item.

Text 2.7

中医的五行学说和阴阳学说一样，同样是指导中医临床工作的。举例来说，如木性条畅，肝气也应舒畅，郁则为病，治以舒肝理气；木能克土，肝病可以犯脾，未犯前，就应当预为防止，已发现脾病时，则宜疏肝健脾；水能生木，所以肝虚的病症，可用滋肾的方法来柔肝；金能克木，则肝旺的症候，可用佐金平肝法。

Transliteration 2.7

Zhōng-yī de wǔ-xíng xué-shuō hé yīn yáng xué-shuō yī-yàng, tóng-yàng shì zhǐ-dǎo zhōng-yī lín-chuáng gōng-zuò de. Jǔ-lì-lái shuō, rú mù xìng tiáo-chàng, gān-qì yě yīng shū-chàng, yù zé wéi bìng, zhì yǐ shū gān lǐ-qì; mù néng kè tǔ, gān-bìng kě-yǐ fàn pí, wèi fàn qián, jiù yīng-dāng yù-wéi fáng-zhǐ, yǐ fā-xiàn pí-bìng shí, zé yí shū-gān jiàn-pí; shuǐ néng shēng mù, suǒ-yǐ gān-xū de bìng-zhèng, kě yòng zī-shèn de fāng-fǎ lái róu-gān; jīn néng kè mù, zé gān-wàng de zhèng-hòu, kě yòng zuǒ jīn píng-gān fǎ.

Vocabulary 2.7

和	hé	with; and
一样	yī-yàng	in the same way
和 ... 一样	hé ... yī-yàng	in the same way as ...
同样	tóng-yàng	likewise
工作	gōng-zuò	work; activity
举例来说	jǔ-lì-lái shuō	to explain by way of example
条畅	tiáo-chàng	pass through; be unimpeded
肝气	gān-qì	liver qi
舒畅	shū-chàng	be unimpeded
郁	yù	depressed; impeded
治	zhì	treat
舒	shū	free; open
理气	lǐ-qì	regulate the (flow of the) qi
肝病	gān-bìng	liver illness
未	wèi	not; not yet
前	qián	before
未 ... 前	wèi ... qián	before ...
犯	fàn	offend; invade
应当	yīng-dāng	should; must
预为	yù-wéi	prepare
防止	fáng-zhǐ	prevent
已	yǐ	already
已 ... 时，则 ...	yǐ ... shí, zé ...	if already ..., then ...
脾病	pí-bìng	spleen illness
宜	yí	should; appropriate
疏肝	shū-gān	clear the liver
健脾	jiàn-pí	strengthen the spleen
肝虚	gān-xū	liver depletion
病症	bìng-zhèng	pathocondition

滋肾	zī-shèn	enrich the kidneys
柔肝	róu-gān	emolliate the liver
肝旺	gān-wàng	liver effulgence
症候	zhèng-hòu	symptoms
佐	zuǒ	assist

Translation 2.7

Both the five phases doctrine and the yinyang doctrine guide the clinical work of Chinese medicine. For example, the nature of wood is to pass through (everything), and hence the qi of the liver should pass through (everything) too. When (the qi of the liver) is impeded (in its flow), that is illness, and (such a condition) is to be treated in that the liver is opened and the qi is regulated. Wood is able to restrain the soil. Hence liver illnesses are able to invade the spleen. As long as such an invasion has not occurred yet, it is necessary to prepare preventive measures. If, though, an illness is discovered in the spleen already, then it is advisable to clear the liver and to strengthen the spleen. Water can engender wood. Hence in case of a pathocondition of liver depletion, it is possible to employ a method to enrich the kidneys to emolliate the liver. Metal can restrain wood. Therefore, in case of symptoms of liver effulgence, it is possible to employ (therapeutic) patterns to assist the metal and balance the liver.

Text 2.8

其它脏病，如肺劳用培土生金法，脾泻用益火培土法，都是按照五行相生，相克的道理处理的。从这些治法的运用上，也可说明一个问题，即中医非但不把内脏孤立起来，而且极其重视内脏之间的密切联系，常常在甲脏有病时，从乙脏或丙脏来进行治疗，因而有"隔一"，"隔二"和"虚则补其母，实则泻其子"等方法。

Transliteration 2.8

Qí-tā zàng-bìng, rú fèi-láo yòng péi-tǔ shēng-jīn fǎ, pí-xiè yòng yì-huǒ péi-tǔ fǎ, dōu-shì àn-zhào wǔ-xíng xiāng-shēng, xiāng-kè de dào-lǐ chǔ-lǐ de. Cóng zhè-xiē zhì-fǎ de yùn-yòng shàng, yě kě shuō-míng yī ge wèn-tí, jí zhōng-yī fēi-dàn bù bǎ nèi-zàng gū-lì qǐ-lái, ér-qiě jí-qí zhòng-shì nèi-zàng zhī-jiān de mì-qiè lián-xì, cháng-cháng zài jiǎ zàng yǒu bìng shí, cóng yǐ zàng huò bǐng zàng lái jìn-xíng zhì-liáo, yīn-ér yǒu "gé yī," "gé èr" hé "xū zé bǔ qí mǔ, shí ze xiè qí zǐ" děng fāng-fǎ.

Vocabulary 2.8

脏病	zàng-bìng	illnesses of the depots
肺劳	fèi-láo	taxation of the lung
培土	péi-tǔ	heap soil
生金	shēng-jīn	generate metal
脾泻	pí-xiè	spleen drainage
益火	yì-huǒ	boost fire
按照	àn-zhào	in accordance with
处理	chǔ-lǐ	deal with; sort out; handle
这些	zhè-xiē	these
治法	zhì-fǎ	therapeutic pattern
从 ... 上	cóng ... shàng	starting from ...; on the basis of
非但 ... 而且	fēi-dàn ... ér-qiě	not only ..., but also
内脏	nèi-zàng	inner depots
孤立	gū-lì	isolate
极其	jí-qí	extremely
重视	zhòng-shì	regard highly; pay attention to
常常	cháng-cháng	often; regularly
在 ... 时	zài ... shí	while; during ...
甲	jiǎ	first (in an enumeration)
乙	yǐ	second (in an enumeration)
丙	bǐng	third (in an enumeration)
进行	jìn-xíng	conduct; carry out
隔	gé	distance; separation
补	bǔ	supplement
其	qí	his; her; its

Translation 2.8

All other illnesses of the depots – as for instance taxation of the lung, in which case a (therapeutic) pattern of heaping the soil and of generating metal is employed, or spleen drainage, in which case a pattern of boosting the fire and heaping the soil is employed, are dealt with in accordance with the principles of mutual engendering and mutual restraint among the five phases. On the basis of an application of these therapeutic patterns it is possible to illustrate one (particular) issue, that is, Chinese medicine not only avoids isolating the individual depots, on the contrary, it pays highest attention to the close relationships among them. When a first depot has an illness, usually a therapy is conducted starting from a second or third depot (in the sequences of mutual engendering or restraint). Hence there are (therapeutic) patterns such as "separated by one[1]" or "separated by two" as well as "in case of depletion supplement the mother; in case of repletion drain its son[2]."

Notes

1 That is, to treat a depot that is separated, in the sequence of mutual engendering or restraint, from the diseased depot by one depot situated in between. For example, wood generates fire, fire generates soil. A treatment "separated by one" is directed at the wood, when the soil is diseased.

2 Wood generates fire. Wood is the mother; fire is the son.

Text 3.1

经络学说也是中医理论体系中重要的组成部分。它为医者必修的一门课程和阴阳，五行学说一样，贯串在中医的生理，病理，诊断，治法，药物等各个方面，并起有重大的作用。经络，直者为经，横者为络，网罗全身，错综联系。它的作用是内属脏腑，外络形体，行气血，营阴阳，濡筋骨，利关节。全身经络，主要的为十二经脉，十二经别，十二经筋和奇经八脉。

Transliteration 3.1

Jīng-luò xué-shuō yě shì zhōng-yī lǐ-lùn tǐ-xì zhōng zhòng-yào de zǔ-chéng bù-fèn. Tā wéi yī-zhě bì xiū de yī mén kè-chéng hé yīn yáng, wǔ-xíng xué-shuō yī-yàng, guàn-chuàn zài zhōng-yī de shēng-lǐ, bìng-lǐ, zhěn-duàn, zhì-fǎ, yào-wù děng gè-ge fāng-miàn, bìng qǐ-yǒu zhòng-dà de zuò-yòng. Jīng-luò, zhí zhě wéi jīng, héng zhě wéi luò, wǎng-luó quán-shēn, cuò-zōng lián-xì. Tā-de zuò-yòng shì nèi shǔ zàng-fǔ, wài luò xíng-tǐ, xíng qì xuè, yíng yīn yáng, rú jīn gǔ, lì guān-jié. Quán-shēn jīng-luò, zhǔ-yào de wéi shí-èr jīng-mài, shí-èr jīng-bié, shí-èr jīng-jīn hé qí-jīng-bā-mài.

Vocabulary 3.1

经络	jīng-luò	conduits and network (vessels)
重要	zhòng-yào	important
组成	zǔ-chéng	constitute; constitutive
部分	bù-fèn	element
组成部分	zǔ-chéng bù-fèn	constitutive element
医者	yī-zhě	physicians
修	xiū	study; care about
门	mén	(numerial for disciplines in science and medicine)
课程	kè-chéng	branch of study; subject
在 ... 的	zài ... de	being in ...
起有	qǐ-yǒu	fulfill
重大	zhòng-dà	important
直	zhí	straight; lengthwise
经	jīng	conduit
横	héng	crosswise
络	luò	network (vessel); enclose
网罗	wǎng-luó	interconnect
全身	quán-shēn	the entire body
错综	cuò-zōng	complicated

它的	tā-de	its (possessive pronoun; genitive singular)
形体	xíng-tǐ	the physical body
营	yíng	nourish
濡	rú	moisten
利	lì	benefit; advantage; (here:) maintain a free movement
关节	guān-jié	joint
十二	shí-èr	twelve
经脉	jīng-mài	conduit vessels
经别	jīng-bié	conduit branches
经筋	jīng-jīn	conduit sinew
奇经八脉	qí-jīng-bā-mài	the eight extraordinary conduit vessels

Translation 3.1

In the theoretical system of Chinese medicine, the doctrine of the conduits and network (vessels) represents an important constitutive element too. It is a subject that must be studied by physicians; in the same way as the yinyang and five phases doctrines, it penetrates all aspects of Chinese medicine, including physiology, pathology, diagnosis, therapy, and pharmaceutics, and it fulfills an important function in all of them alike. The conduits and network (vessels) – those (running) straight (through the body) are the conduits, and those (running) crosswise are the network (vessels) – interconnect the entire body, (generating) complicated relationships. Their functions are (the following). In the interior, they connect with the depots and palaces; in the exterior, they enclose the physical body. They transmit the qi and the blood; they nourish the yin and the yang (regions); they moisten sinews and bones; and they ensure the movement of the joints. Of the conduits and network (vessels) of the entire body, the twelve conduit vessels, the twelve conduit branches, the twelve conduit sinews, and the eight extraordinary conduit vessels are the important ones.

Text 3.2

其中十二经脉分为六支阳经，六支阴经，逐经相传，循行脏腑，头面，四肢；经别是十二经脉的别出，在阳经和阴经之间构成表里配合，着重于深部的联系；经筋是起于肢末，行于体表，着重于浅部的联系；奇经八脉则为调节十二经脉的。

Transliteration 3.2

Qí-zhōng shí-èr jīng-mài fēn-wéi liù zhī yáng-jīng, liù zhī yīn-jīng, zhú-jīng xiāng-chuán, xún-xíng zàng-fǔ, tóu-miàn, sì-zhī; jīng-bié shì shí-èr jīng-mài de bié-chū, zài yáng-jīng hé yīn-jīng zhī-jiān gòu-chéng biǎo lǐ pèi-hé, zhuó-zhòng yú shēn-bù de lián-xì; jīng-jīn shì qǐ yú zhī-mò, xíng-yú tǐ-biǎo, zhuó-zhòng yú qiǎn-bù de lián-xì; qí-jīng-bā-mài zé wéi tiáo-jié shí-èr jīng-mài de.

Vocabulary 3.2

其中	qí-zhōng	among them
分为	fēn-wéi	divide into
支	zhī	(measure word for conduits, branches, and sidelines)
阳经	yáng-jīng	yang conduits
阴经	yīn-jīng	yin conduits
逐	zhú	follow
逐经	zhú-jīng	one conduit after another
传	chuán	transmit
相传	xiāng-chuán	transmit each other
循行	xún-xíng	penetrate; pass through
头面	tóu-miàn	head and face
肢	zhī	limb; extremity
四肢	sì-zhī	the four limbs
别出	bié-chū	offshoots
配合	pèi-hé	combination; matching
着重	zhuó-zhòng	emphasize
深部	shēn-bù	deep-lying regions
是	shì	(particle emphasizing the statement of the following verb)
末	mò	end
肢末	zhī-mò	the ends of the limbs
行于	xíng-yú	pass through
浅部	qiǎn-bù	surface region
调节	tiáo-jié	regulate

Translation 3.2

Among these (conduits and network vessels) the twelve conduit vessels are divided into six yang conduits and six yin conduits. The conduits transmit (their contents) among each other, and they pass through the depots and palaces, the head and the face, and the four limbs. The conduit branches are offshoots of the twelve conduit vessels. Situated between the yang conduits and the yin conduits, they fashion a matching of the exterior with the interior, with an emphasis on connections with/of the deep-lying regions. The conduit sinews arise from the ends of the limbs. They pass through the body's exterior, with an emphasis on the connections in the surface regions. The eight extraordinary conduit vessels serve to regulate the (contents of the) twelve conduit vessels.

Text 3.3

所以经脉是气血运行必由的通路，贯串在人体内外，上下，左右，前后，从而将人体各部分包括五脏，六腑，头面，躯干，四肢，九窍等，联系成为有机的统一整体。并由于经络互相衔接，由阴入阳，由阳入阴，从里走表，从表走里，自上而下，自下而上，气血流行，循环不息，所谓阴阳相随，内外相贯，如环无端。

Transliteration 3.3

Suǒ-yǐ jīng-mài shì qì xuè yùn-xíng bì-yóu de tōng-lù, guàn-chuàn zài rén-tǐ nèi wài, shàng xià, zuǒ yòu, qián hòu, cóng-ér jiāng rén-tǐ gè bù-fèn bāo-kuò wǔ-zàng, liù-fǔ, tóu-miàn, qū-gàn, sì-zhī, jiǔ-qiào děng, lián-xì chéng-wéi yǒu-jī de tǒng-yī zhěng-tǐ. Bìng yóu-yú jīng-luò hù-xiāng xián-jiē, yóu yīn rù yáng, yóu yáng rù yīn, cóng lǐ zǒu biǎo, cóng biǎo zǒu lǐ, zì shàng ér xià, zì xià ér shàng, qì xuè liú-xíng, xún huán bù xī, suǒ-wèi yīn yáng xiāng-suí, nèi wài xiāng-guàn, rú huán wú duān.

Vocabulary 3.3

运行	yùn-xíng	transmission
必由	bì-yóu	essential; necessary
通路	tōng-lù	pathway; thoroughfare
左	zuǒ	left
右	yòu	right
后	hòu	back; behind
体	tǐ	substance; body
躯干	qū-gàn	trunk
九窍	jiǔ-qiào	the nine orifices
有机	yǒu-jī	organic
整体	zhěng-tǐ	whole
由于	yóu-yú	because of ...
互相	hù-xiāng	each other
衔接	xián-jiē	link
由	yóu	from; take its origin in
入	rù	enter
走	zǒu	go; move
自	zì	from
自上而下	zì shàng ér xià	from above downwards
流行	liú-xíng	flow
循	xún	follow; along with
环	huán	circle
息	xī	stop; break
循环不息	xún huán bù xī	circular flow without pause
所谓	suǒ-wèi	so-called
相随	xiāng-suí	follow each other
相贯	xiāng-guàn	linked to each other
如环无端	rú huán wú duān	like a ring without end

Translation 3.3

Hence the conduit vessels are essential pathways for the transmission of qi and blood. They penetrate the human body's inner and outer, upper and lower, left and right, front and back (regions), and in that they connect all parts of the human body including the five depots, the six palaces, the head and the face, the trunk, the four limbs, and the nine orifices they create an integrated organic whole. Also, because the conduits and the network (vessels) are linked up with each other, (and because) from the yin they enter the yang, from the yang they enter the yin, from the interior they move to the exterior, from the exterior they move to the interior, from above they descend, and from below they rise, the flow of qi and blood is a circulation without pause. (This is) what is called "yin and yang follow each other," "inner and outer are linked to each other," and (the circulation of the qi is) "like a ring without end."

Text 3.4

人体生理功能，是以五脏六腑为主，但使人体内外，上下保持着平衡的协调，进行有机的整体活动，则经络起有重要的作用。经络学说，是前人在长时期的临症实践中根据无数病例治疗效果的分析研究而形成的。故用经络来分析症候，也能作为辨症论治的准则之一。

Transliteration 3.4

Rén-tǐ shēng-lǐ gōng-néng, shì yǐ wǔ-zàng liù-fǔ wéi-zhǔ, dàn shǐ rén-tǐ nèi wài, shàng xià bǎo-chí zhe píng-héng de xié-tiáo, jìn-xíng yǒu-jī de zhěng-tǐ huó-dòng, zé jīng-luò qǐ yǒu zhòng-yào de zuò-yòng. Jīng-luò xué-shuō, shì qián-rén zài cháng-shí-qī de lín-zhèng shí-jiàn zhōng gēn-jù wú-shù bìng-lì zhì-liáo xiào-guǒ de fēn-xī yán-jiū ér xíng-chéng de. Gù yòng jīng-luò lái fēn-xī zhèng-hòu, yě néng zuò-wéi biàn-zhèng lùn-zhì de zhǔn-zé zhī-yī.

Vocabulary 3.4

以 ... 为主	yǐ ... wéi-zhǔ	rest mainly on ...
保持	bǎo-chí	maintain
协调	xié-tiáo	harmonize; harmony
活动	huó-dòng	activity
长时期	cháng-shí-qī	long-term
无数	wú-shù	innumerable; countless
病例	bìng-lì	a case of illness
效果	xiào-guǒ	result
研究	yán-jiū	research
形成	xíng-chéng	form
作为	zuò-wéi	consider as ...
辨	biàn	differentiate; differentiation
论	lùn	determine; discuss
辨症论治	biàn-zhèng-lùn-zhì	determine a therapy on the basis of a differentiation of (a patient's) pathoconditions
准则	zhǔn-zé	criterion
之一	zhī-yī	one of ...

Translation 3.4

The human body's physiological functions rest mainly on the five depots and six palaces. However, when it comes to maintaining a balanced harmony in the body's inner and outer, upper and lower (sections), and to carry out activities (essential) for an organic whole, then the conduits and network (vessels) play an important role. The doctrine of the conduits and network (vessels) was formed by people in former times in the course of long-term clinical practice on the basis of analytical research of the results of the treatment of innumerable cases of illness. Hence to employ (the doctrine of) the conduits and network (vessels) to analyze the signs of an illness may also be considered as one of the criteria for determining a therapy on the basis of a differentiation of (a patient's) pathoconditions.

Text 3.5

一般外邪的传变，大多通过经络由表入里，由浅入深。如以真中风病来说，轻者中络，症见肌肤麻木，口眼歪斜；稍重中经，症见左瘫右痪，身重不胜；再重则中腑，中脏，症见口噤，舌强，神昏不醒，便溺或阻或遗。又如自内脏发生的疾病，同样会在所属经络反映出来，如肺，心有邪，其气留于两肘，肝有邪其气留于两胁，脾有邪其气留于两髀，肾有邪其气留于两腘。气留则痛，临症上常可遇到。

Transliteration 3.5

Yī-bān wài-xié de chuán-biàn, dà-duō tōng-guò jīng-luò yóu biǎo rù lǐ, yóu qiǎn rù shēn. Rú yǐ zhēn zhòng-fēng bìng lái shuō, qīng zhě zhòng luò, zhèng jiàn jī-fū má-mù, kǒu yǎn wāi-xié; shāo zhòng zhòng jīng, zhèng jiàn zuǒ-tān-yòu-huàn, shēn zhòng bù shèng; zài zhòng zé zhòng fǔ, zhòng zàng, zhèng jiàn kǒu-jìn, shé-jiàng, shén hūn bù-xǐng, biàn-niào huò zǔ huò yí. Yòu rú zì nèi-zàng fā-shēng de jí-bìng, tóng-yàng huì zài suǒ-shǔ jīng-luò fǎn-yìng chū-lái, rú fèi, xīn yǒu xié, qí qì liú yú liǎng zhǒu, gān yǒu xié qí qì liú yú liǎng xié, pí yǒu xié qí qì liú yú liǎng bì, shèn yǒu xié qí qì liú yú liǎng guó. Qì liú zé tòng, lín-zhèng shàng cháng kě yù-dào.

Vocabulary 3.5

外邪	wài-xié	external evil
传变	chuán-biàn	transmission and change
大多	dà-duō	mostly; in general
浅	qiǎn	shallow; superficial
深	shēn	deep
真	zhēn	true
中	zhòng	strike
中风	zhòng-fēng	struck by wind
轻	qīng	light; minor
肌肤	jī-fū	the (human) skin
麻木	má-mù	insensitivity
眼	yǎn	eye
歪斜	wāi-xié	wry
稍	shāo	few; little
重	zhòng	heavy; serious
左瘫右痪	zuǒ-tān-yòu-huàn	left and right side paralysis
口噤	kǒu-jìn	trismus
强	jiàng	stiff
舌强	shé-jiàng	stiffness of the tongue
神	shén	spirit

昏	hūn	confused
醒	xǐng	wake up
不醒	bù-xǐng	unconscious
便溺	biàn-niào	urine
阻	zǔ	blocked
遗	yí	uncontrolled flow
发生	fā-shēng	develop; generate
疾病	jí-bìng	illness
会	huì	can; be able to
所属	suǒ-shǔ	associated; belonging
反映	fǎn-yìng	appear; be reflected in
邪	xié	evil
留	liú	remain
肘	zhǒu	ellbow
胁	xié	flank
髀	bì	upper thigh
腘	guó	popliteal fossa
痛	tòng	pain
常	cháng	often; regular
遇到	yù-dào	encounter

Translation 3.5

In general, transmissions and changes of external evils occur mostly through the conduits and network (vessels) from the exterior into the interior, and from the superficial into the deep-lying (regions of the body). To take the illness of true wind stroke as an example, a minor (stroke) hits the network (vessels), with dermal insensitivity, and a wry mouth and eyes appearing as pathoconditions. A slightly more serious (stroke) hits the conduits, with left and right side paralysis, and an insurmountable (feeling of a) heavy body appearing as pathoconditions. Even more serious (strokes) hit the palaces, and they hit the depots, with trismus, stiffness of the tongue, loss of consciousness, and stoppage or uncontrolled flow of stools and urine appearing as pathoconditions. Also, illnesses that have developed from the inner depots may equally appear in those conduits and network (vessels these depots are) associated with. For example, when the lung or the heart have an evil, its qi settles in the elbows; when the liver has an evil, its qi settles in the two flanks; when the spleen has an evil, its qi settles in the two upper thighs; and when the kidneys have an evil its qi settles in the two popliteal fossae. When qi settles (at some location), then there is pain. That can be encountered often in clinical reality.

Text 3.6

在临症治疗上，经络也是重要依据之一。大家熟悉的针刺手上合谷穴，能治龈肿齿痛；刺足三里穴，能治胃病，这些都是通过经络所起的作用。此外，经络与处方用药也有关系，如中药学上将药物的主治功能分属十二经，见哪一经病用哪一类药。

Transliteration 3.6

Zài lín-zhèng zhì-liáo shàng, jīng-luò yě shì zhòng-yào yī-jù zhī-yī. Dà-jiā shú-xī de zhēn-cì shǒu shàng hé-gǔ xué, néng zhì yín-zhǒng chǐ-tòng; cì zú-sān-lǐ xué, néng zhì wèi-bìng, zhè-xiē dōu-shì tōng-guò jīng-luò suǒ qǐ de zuò-yòng. Cǐ-wài, jīng-luò yǔ chǔ-fāng yòng-yào yě yǒu guān-xi, rú zhōng-yào-xué shàng jiāng yào-wù de zhǔ zhì gōng-néng fēn-shǔ shí-èr jīng, jiàn nǎ-yī jīng-bìng yòng nǎ-yī lèi yào.

Vocabulary 3.6

依据	yī-jù	foundation
大家	dà-jiā	all; everybody
熟悉	shú-xī	be familiar with
针	zhēn	needle
刺	cì	prick
针刺	zhēn-cì	needling
手	shǒu	hand
合谷	hé-gǔ	the he-gu (hole)
龈	yín	gums
龈肿	yín-zhǒng	swollen gums
齿	chǐ	tooth
齿痛	chǐ-tòng	toothache
足三里	zú-sān-lǐ	the leg san-li (hole)
穴	xué	hole; opening
胃病	wèi-bìng	stomach ailment
处方	chǔ-fāng	prescription; write a prescription
中药学	zhōng-yào-xué	Chinese pharmaceutics
分属	fēn-shǔ	assign
哪一	nǎ-yī	which
类	lèi	type; category

Translation 3.6

In clinical therapy, the conduits and network (vessels) constitute an important foundation too. The well-known needling of the he-gu hole on the hand can heal swollen gums and toothache; needling of the leg san-li hole can treat stomach ailments. All these effects are stimulated through the conduits and network (vessels). In addition, the conduits and network (vessels) are also related to the writing of prescriptions and the application of drugs. For example, in Chinese pharmaceutics, the major therapeutic functions of drugs are assigned to the twelve conduits; if an illness is observed in a particular conduit, a particular drug is employed accordingly.

Text 3.7

象麻黄入太阳经，葛根入阳明经，柴胡入少阳经。以上三药均能治疗风寒头痛，如痛在后脑及项者，属太阳经，用麻黄；痛在前额及眉棱骨者，属阳明经，用葛根；痛在头之两侧或一侧者，属少阳经，用柴胡。其它尚有一些药常用于某种病症，成为某种病的主药，如辛夷用于鼻塞，狗脊用于背脊疼痛等，都是从分经上来的。

Transliteration 3.7

Xiàng má-huáng rù tài-yáng-jīng, gé-gēn rù yáng-míng-jīng, chái-hú rù shào-yáng-jīng. Yǐ-shàng sān yào jūn néng zhì-liáo fēng-hán tóu-tòng, rú tòng zài hòu-nǎo jí xiàng zhě, shǔ tài-yáng-jīng, yòng má-huáng; tòng zài qián-é jí méi-léng-gǔ zhě, shǔ yáng-míng-jīng, yòng gé-gēn; tòng zài tóu zhī liǎng cè huò yī cè zhě, shǔ shào-yáng-jīng, yòng chái-hú. Qí-tā shàng yǒu yī-xiē yào cháng yòng yú mǒu-zhǒng bìng-zhèng, chéng-wéi mǒu-zhǒng bìng de zhǔ-yào, rú xīn-yí yòng yú bí-sè, gǒu-jǐ yòng yú bèi-jǐ téng-tòng děng, dōu-shì cóng fēn jīng shàng lái de.

Vocabulary 3.7

象	xiàng	for example
麻黄	má-huáng	(drug name) Ephedra sinica Staph.
太阳经	tài-yáng-jīng	major yang conduit
葛根	gé-gēn	(drug name) Pueraria lobata (Willd.) Ohwi.
阳明经	yáng-míng-jīng	yang brilliance conduit
柴胡	chái-hú	(drug name) Bupleurum chinense D C.
少阳经	shào-yáng-jīng	minor yang conduit
以上	yǐ-shàng	above
三	sān	three
风寒	fēng-hán	wind cold
头	tóu	head
头痛	tóu-tòng	headache
后脑	hòu-nǎo	metencephalon
及	jí	and
项	xiàng	nape
前额	qián-é	forehead
眉棱骨	méi-léng-gǔ	superciliary ridge
尚	shàng	still
一些	yī-xiē	some
主药	zhǔ-yào	master drug
辛夷	xīn-yí	(drug name) Magnolia liliflora Desr.
鼻塞	bí-sè	nasal blockage

狗脊	gǒu-jǐ	(drug name) Cibotium barometz (L.) J. Sm.
背脊	bèi-jǐ	back
疼痛	téng-tòng	pain

Translation 3.7

For example, mahuang enters the major yang conduit; gegen enters the yang brilliance conduit; chaihu enters the minor yang conduit. These three drugs all alike can treat a headache caused by wind and cold. However, if the pain occurs in the metencephalon or in the nape, it is associated with the major yang conduit, and mahuang is employed (for treatment). If the pain occurs in the forehead and in the superciliary ridge, it is associated with the yang brilliance conduit, and gegen is employed (for treatment). If the pain occurs on both sides of the head, or on only one side, it is associated with the minor yang conduit, and chaihu is employed (for treatment). In addition, there are some drugs which are often used against the pathoconditions of specific illnesses, and which represent master drugs of these specific illnesses. For example, xinyi is used against nasal blockages, and gouji is used against back pain. All (these effects) have come about through different conduits.

Text 3.8

一般认为经络学说专门指导针灸治疗的理论根据，这是不全面的。中医无论内科，外科以及妇，幼，推拿，正骨各科，从来没有脱离以经络学说为指导的范畴。经络学说的重要性，在长期实践中已经证明其实际价值，近来通过中西医密切合作，在实验研究中也初步证实了好些问题。如针刺委中，内庭，足三里等穴后，胃的蠕动，胃张力及排空时间均有显明变化；针刺合谷，三阴交等穴，可使子宫收缩加强和间隔缩短。这些不仅说明了针刺对内脏活动的影响，也说明了经络与脏器的关系，值得注意。

Transliteration 3.8

Yī-bān rèn-wéi jīng-luò xué-shuō zhuān-mén zhǐ-dǎo zhēn-jiǔ zhì-liáo de lǐ-lùn gēn-jù, zhè shì bù quán-miàn de. Zhōng-yī wú-lùn nèi-kē, wài-kē yǐ-jí fù, yòu, tuī-ná, zhèng-gǔ gè kē, cóng lái méi-yǒu tuō-lí yǐ jīng-luò xué-shuō wéi zhǐ-dǎo de fàn-chóu. Jīng-luò xué-shuō de zhòng-yào-xìng, zài cháng-qī shí-jiàn zhōng yǐ-jīng zhèng-míng qí shí-jì jià-zhí, jìn-lái tōng-guò zhōng-xī-yī mì-qiè hé-zuò, zài shí-yàn yán-jiū zhōng yě chū-bù zhèng-shí le hǎo-xiē wèn-tí. Rú zhēn-cì wěi-zhōng, nèi-tíng, zú-sān-lǐ děng xué hòu, wèi de rú-dòng, wèi zhāng-lì jí pái-kōng shí-jiān jūn yǒu xiǎn-míng biàn-huà; zhēn-cì hé-gǔ, sān-yīn-jiāo děng xué, kě shǐ zǐ-gōng shōu-suō jiā-qiáng hé jiàn-gé suō-duǎn. Zhè-xiē bù-jǐn shuō-míng le zhēn-cì duì nèi-zàng huó-dòng de yǐng-xiǎng, yě shuō-míng le jīng-luò yǔ zàng-qì de guān-xi, zhí-de zhù-yì.

Vocabulary 3.8

专门	zhuān-mén	exclusively; specialized
灸	jiǔ	moxa
针灸	zhēn-jiǔ	acupuncture and moxa therapy
不全面	bù quán-miàn	incomplete
无论	wú-lùn	regardless whether ...
内科	nèi-kē	internal medicine
妇	fù	woman
幼	yòu	child; youth
推拿	tuī-ná	manual therapy

正骨	zhèng-gǔ	chiropractice; bone correcting
没有	méi-yǒu	does not exist; there is no ...
脱离	tuō-lí	disassociate from
范畴	fàn-chóu	realm; category
重要性	zhòng-yào-xìng	importance
长期	cháng-qī	longtime
已经	yǐ-jīng	already
证明	zhèng-míng	demonstrate
价值	jià-zhí	value
近来	jìn-lái	recently
中西医	zhōng-xī-yī	Chinese and Western medicine
合作	hé-zuò	cooperation
实验	shí-yàn	experiment; experimental
初步	chū-bù	preliminary
证实	zhèng-shí	evidence
好些	hǎo-xiē	many
委中	wěi-zhōng	wei-zhong (hole)
内庭	nèi-tíng	nei-ting (hole)
蠕动	rú-dòng	peristalsis
张力	zhāng-lì	tension
排空	pái-kōng	evacuation
时间	shí-jiān	time
显明	xiǎn-míng	significant
三阴交	sān-yīn-jiāo	san-yin-jiao (hole)
子宫	zǐ-gōng	uterus
收缩	shōu-suō	contraction
加强	jiā-qiáng	strengthen
间隔	jiàn-gé	interval
缩短	suō-duǎn	shorten
不仅	bù-jǐn	not only
对	duì	on; at
影响	yǐng-xiǎng	influence
脏器	zàng-qì	depot organ
值得	zhí-de	be worth
注意	zhù-yì	pay attention

Translation 3.8

It is generally assumed that the doctrine of the conduits and network (vessels) exclusively guides the theoretical basis of acupuncture and moxa therapy. (However), there is more to it. Chinese medicine has never disassociated itself in any special field – no matter whether this is internal medicine, external medicine, gynecology and pediatrics, manual therapy or chiropractice – from a realm (of thought) viewing the doctrine of the conduits and network (vessels) as guiding category. As for the importance of the doctrine of the conduits and network (vessels), (this doctrine) has already demonstrated its practical value in the course of its longtime application. More recently, in the process of a close cooperation between Chinese and Western medicine, and in experimental research, (the doctrine of the conduits and network vessels) has provided preliminary evidence to many questions. For example, following a needling of the wei-zhong, the nei-ting, and the leg san-li holes, the gastric peristalsis, as well as gastric tension and evacuation time all underwent significant changes. Needling the he-gu and san-yin-jiao holes can cause a strengthening of uterine contractions as well as a shortening of the invertals (in between these contractions). These (effects) do not only explain the influence of needling on the activities of the internal depots, they also explain the relationships between the conduits and network (vessels on the one side) and the depot organs (on the other). This is worth (our) attention.

Text 4.1

五脏是心，肝，脾，肺，肾，六腑是胆，胃，小肠，大肠，膀胱和三焦，五脏中还有心包络，为心的外卫，也有把它独立起来，与五脏并列，称为六脏，惟心包络的功能和病变总是与心脏相一致的。脏和腑俱为内脏，其区别是：五脏藏精气而不泻，六腑传化物而不藏。凡具有出纳转输，传化水谷功能的脏器，归属于腑；没有直接传化水谷而具有贮藏精气功能的脏器，归属于脏。

cháng, ...
de wài-wèi, ...
zàng, wéi xīn-bāo-luò ...
xiāng yī-zhì de. Zàng hé fǔ ...
jīng-qì ér bù xiè, liù-fǔ chuán-huà ...
zhuǎn-shū, chuán-huà shuǐ-gǔ gōng-néng de ...
zhí-jiē chuán-huà shuǐ-gǔ ér jù-yǒu zhù-cáng jīng-qì ...
guī-shǔ yú zàng.

shì dǎn, wèi, xiǎo-cháng, dà-
...ái-yǒu xīn-bāo-luò, wéi xīn
...bìng liè, chēng-wéi liù-
...ng shì yǔ xīn-zàng
... wǔ-zàng cáng
...-yǒu chū-nà
... méi-yǒu
...ng-qì,

Vocabulary 4.1

胆	dǎn	gallbladder
小肠	xiǎo-cháng	small intestine
大肠	dà-cháng	large intestine
膀胱	páng-guāng	urinary bladder
三焦	sān-jiāo	triple burner
心包络	xīn-bāo-luò	heart-enclosing-network
外卫	wài-wèi	outer protection
独立	dú-lì	independent
起来	qǐ-lái	raise; mention
并	bìng	together
列	liè	list; enumerate
称为	chēng-wéi	call
惟	wéi	however; only
总	zǒng	always
心脏	xīn-zàng	heart
与 ... 相	yǔ ... xiāng	in comparison with
一致	yī-zhì	identical
俱	jù	all
传化	chuán-huà	transmit and transform
物	wù	item; thing; substance

凡 fán
出纳 chū-n... ...and taking in; input
...output
转输 ...orward; transfer; pass along
水谷 water and grain; liquid and solid food
归属 belong
贮藏 ...ng store

...ation 4.1

The five depots are the heart, the liver, the spleen, the lung, and the kidneys; the six palaces include the gallbladder, the stomach, the small intestine, the large intestine, the bladder, and the triple burner. In addition, there is the heart-enclosing-network among the five depots; it is the outer protection of the heart. It may also be referred to individually, and is listed then together with the five depots which are then called six depots, even though the functions and the pathological changes of the heart-enclosing-network are entirely the same as those of the heart. The depots and the palaces together are the inner depots. Their difference is: the five depots store the essential qi and do not drain; the six palaces transmit and transform things but do not store. All those depot organs with functions of a putting out, taking in, and passing on, and of transmitting and transforming water and grain, belong to the palaces. Those depot organs that have no functions of directly transmitting and transforming liquid and solid food, and that serve to store essential qi, belong to the depots.

病邪	bìng-xié	pathogenic evil
侵犯	qīn-fàn	intrude
出现	chū-xiàn	let appear; bring forth
心悸	xīn-jì	palpitations
惊惕	jīng-tì	shock
失眠	shī-mián	insomnia
善忘	shàn-wàng	forgetfulness
笑	xiào	laughter
失常	shī-cháng	irregular
谵语	zhān-yǔ	wild talk
神识	shén-zhì	mental
昏迷	hūn-mí	confusion
不仅 ... 并 ...	bù-jǐn ... bìng ...	not only ..., but also ...
无以	wú-yǐ	have nothing to ...
自	zì	self
自主	zì-zhǔ	self-control
紊乱	wěn-luàn	disorder
谋虑	móu-lǜ	plotting and planning
刚强	gāng-qiáng	strength
将军	jiāng-jūn	general; troop leader
称号	chēng-hào	title; designation
受到	shòu-dào	receive
精神	jīng-shén	spirit; mental
往往	wǎng-wǎng	often
正常	zhèng-cháng	normal
恼怒	nǎo-nù	anger
胀	zhàng	distension
头胀	tóu-zhàng	a feeling of heaviness in the head
甚至	shèn-zhì	even; possibly going as far as to
火气	huǒ-qì	fire qi
上逆	shàng-nì	rise
吐	tù	spit; vomit
女子	nǚ-zǐ	female; woman
先天	xiān-tiān	earlier dependence

生殖	shēng-zhí	reproduction
意思	yì-si	meaning
调	tiáo	regulate
经	jīng	monthly period
种子	zhòng-zǐ	fertility
肝脏	gān-zàng	liver

Translation 4.2

1. The heart: the heart generates the blood, and it is responsible for storing the spirit. It is the ruler of the vital activities of the human body. If the heart itself has a problem, either because it received an emotional stimulus, or because of an intrusion of a pathological evil – it can let pathoconditions appear such as palpitations, shock, and insomnia, or forgetfulness, and irregular joy and laughter, or wild talk and mental confusion. Once the heart has undergone a pathological change, it will not only lose its self-control, it can also influence the activities of other depots and palaces, and let them develop disorder.

2. The liver: The liver stores the blood, and it is responsible for plotting and pondering. The nature of the liver is strength; hence it is also called "general." Mental stimuli often influence its normal functions, and bring about pathoconditions such as anger, or a feeling of heaviness in the head. This may go so far that fire qi rises and causes bloodspitting. In addition, the liver represents the "earlier dependence[1]" of women [that means, it has reproductive functions]. Hence a therapy directed at the liver should be emphasized if it is intended to regulate the monthly period or enhance the fertiliy (of females).

Note

1 The "earlier dependence" refers to all the factors enabling and forming human life between conception and birth. In general the "kidneys" are considered "the source of the earlier dependence."

3. 脾：脾统血，主运化。维持生命的力量主要是营养，脾能消化水谷，把食物的精华运输到全身，故被称为"后天"之本。倘脾的运化能力不足，则食后作胀，因而引起肌肉消瘦，精神疲乏。脾又主运化水湿，水湿停滞的症状，如肌肤浮肿，大便泄泻，大多由于脾弱所致，因此利湿常用健脾方法。

4. 肺：肺主气，司清肃。肺气不降，最易引起咳嗽，气喘，在虚症的情况下，又常见少气，言语低怯无力。肺对于心脏所主的血液循行，有调节作用，前人为了形容两者间的密切关系，曾把心脏称作君主，肺脏称作相傅。

Transliteration 4.3

3. Pí: pí tǒng xuè, zhǔ yùn huà. Wéi-chí shēng-mìng de lì-liang zhǔ-yào shì yíng-yǎng, pí néng xiāo-huà shuǐ-gǔ, bǎ shí-wù de jīng-huá yùn-shū dào quán-shēn, gù bèi chēng-wéi “hòu-tiān” zhī běn. Tǎng pí de yùn huà néng-lì bù-zú, zé shí hòu zuò zhàng, yīn-ér yǐn-qǐ jī-ròu-xiāo-shòu, jīng-shén pí-fá. Pí yòu zhǔ yùn huà shuǐ-shī, shuǐ-shī tíng-zhì de zhèng-zhuàng, rú jī-fū fú-zhǒng, dà-biàn xiè-xiè, dà-duō yóu-yú pí ruò suǒ-zhì, yīn-cǐ lì-shī cháng-yòng jiàn-pí fāng-fǎ.

4. Fèi: fèi zhǔ qì, sī qīng sù. Fèi-qì bù jiàng, zuì yì yǐn-qǐ ké-sòu, qì-chuǎn, zài xū-zhèng de qíng-kuàng xià, yòu cháng jiàn shǎo-qì, yán-yǔ dī-qiè wú-lì. Fèi duì-yú xīn-zàng suǒ zhǔ de xuè-yè xún-xíng, yǒu tiáo-jié zuò-yòng, qián-rén wéi le xíng-róng liǎng zhě jiān de mì-qiè guān-xi, céng bǎ xīn-zàng chēng-zuò jūn-zhǔ, fèi-zàng chēng-zuò xiàng-fu.

Vocabulary 4.3

统	tǒng	govern
运	yùn	transport
力量	lì-liang	strength
营养	yíng-yǎng	nourishment
食物	shí-wù	food

精华	jīng-huá	essence
运输	yùn-shū	transport
到	dào	to
被	bèi	(passive pronoun)
后天	hòu-tiān	the later dependence
倘…则	tǎng ... zé	if ..., then
食	shí	food; meal
作	zuò	make
因而	yīn-ér	hence
肌肉消瘦	jī-ròu-xiāo-shòu	emaciation
疲乏	pí-fá	fatigue
水湿	shuǐ-shī	liquid
停滞	tíng-zhì	stagnate
浮肿	fú-zhǒng	edema
大便	dà-biàn	stool
泄泻	xiè-xiè	diarrhea
…所致	... suǒ-zhì	be caused by ...
利湿	lì-shī	make liquid flow off
常用	cháng-yòng	employ often
司	sī	regulate
清	qīng	clear
肃	sù	lofty
肺气	fèi-qì	lung qi
最	zuì	very; extreme
易	yì	easy
咳嗽	ké-sòu	cough
气喘	qì-chuǎn	panting
虚症	xū-zhèng	pathocondition of depletion
言语	yán-yǔ	speech
低怯	dī-qiè	faint
无力	wú-lì	powerless; weak
对于	duì-yú	on
形容	xíng-róng	describe
曾	céng	once; before
君主	jūn-zhǔ	lord

肺脏	fèi-zàng	lung
相傅	xiàng-fù	minister

Translation 4.3

3. The spleen: The spleen governs the blood; it is responsible for transport and transformation. Nourishment is most important for the maintenance of vital strength. The spleen is able to digest liquid and solid food, and to transport the essence of food throughout the entire body. Hence it is called the basis of the "later dependence.[1]" When the power of the spleen to transport and to transform is insufficient, this will cause distention after the meals, and hence will lead to emaciation and mental fatigue. The spleen is also responsible for transporting and transforming liquids. Pathomanifestations of liquid-stagnation, such as dermal edema and diarrhea, emerge mostly from splenic weakness. Hence (therapeutic) methods of strengthening the spleen are often employed to cause the dampness to flow off.

4. The lung: The lung rules the qi; it controls the clear and lofty. If the lung qi fails to descend, this will most easily lead to coughing and panting. In case of pathoconditions of depletion, diminished qi is often witnessed, as well as faint and powerless speech. The lung has a regulative effect on the movement of the blood which is ruled by the heart. To describe the close relationship between the two, the people in former times called the heart "lord" and the lung "minister."

Note

1 The "later dependence" refers to the means of maintaining human life subsequent to birth. These are especially food and beverages.

Text 4.4

5. 肾：肾藏精，主作强。肾脏对于人的精力充沛起有积极作用，肾虚则脑转，耳鸣，目无所见，腰痛，胫酸，懈怠思卧等症均起。肾为男子的"先天"，与女子以肝为先天的意义相同，即指生殖功能而言。故性欲衰退及滑精，早泄等症，都从肾脏治疗。肾与其它内脏有一不同的特点，即肾有两枚，左者为肾，右者为命门，肾主阴，命门主阳，故肾又有"水火之脏"之称。

Transliteration 4.4

5. Shèn: shèn cáng jīng, zhǔ zuò qiáng. Shèn-zàng duì-yú rén de jīng-lì chōng-pèi qǐ yǒu jī-jí zuò-yòng, shèn-xū zé nǎo-zhuàn, ěr-míng, mù-wú-suǒ-jiàn, yāo-tòng, jìng-suān, xiè-dài sī-wò děng zhèng jūn qǐ. Shèn wéi nán-zǐ de "xiān-tiān," yǔ nǚ-zǐ yǐ gān wéi xiān-tiān de yì-yì xiāng-tóng, jí zhǐ shēng-zhí gōng-néng ér yán. Gù xìng-yù shuāi-tuì jí huá-jīng, zǎo-xiè děng zhèng, dōu cóng shèn-zàng zhì-liáo. Shèn yǔ qí-tā nèi-zàng yǒu yī bù-tóng de tè-diǎn, jí shèn yǒu liǎng méi, zuǒ zhě wéi shèn, yòu zhě wéi mìng-mén, shèn zhǔ yīn, mìng-mén zhǔ yáng, gù shèn yòu yǒu "shuǐ huǒ zhī zàng" zhī chēng.

Vocabulary 4.4

强	qiáng	strong; strength
肾脏	shèn-zàng	kidneys
精力充沛	jīng-lì chōng-pèi	vigor
积极	jī-jí	positive
肾虚	shèn-xū	kidney depletion
脑转	nǎo-zhuàn	spinning head; dizziness
耳鸣	ěr-míng	ringing in the ears
目无所见	mù-wú-suǒ-jiàn	impaired vision
腰痛	yāo-tòng	lumbago
胫酸	jìng-suān	pain in the lower leg
懈怠	xiè-dài	sluggishness
思卧	sī-wò	sleepiness
男子	nán-zǐ	male
相同	xiāng-tóng	be mutually identical
与 ... 相同	yǔ ... xiāng-tóng	identical with ...; correspond to each other
言	yán	speak; refer to
指 ... 而言	zhǐ ... ér yán	refer to
性欲	xìng-yù	libido
衰退	shuāi-tuì	weaken

滑精	huá-jīng	involuntary seminal efflux
早泄	zǎo-xiè	premature ejaculation
特点	tè-diǎn	characteristic
枚	méi	(measure word for flat objects)
命门	mìng-mén	gate of life
称	chēng	designate; call

Translation 4.4

5. The kidneys: The kidneys store the essence; they are responsible for generating strength. The kidneys play a positive part regarding the vigor of man. When the kidneys are depleted, pathoconditions such as dizziness, ringing in the ears, impaired vision, lumbago, pain in the lower leg, sluggishness, and sleepiness all emerge. The kidneys represent the "earlier dependence" in males – the meaning (of this expression) is identical with considering the liver as the earlier dependence in females, that is, it refers to reproductive functions. Hence pathoconditions such as failing sexual desires and involuntary seminal efflux, as well as premature ejaculation, are treated through the kidneys. The kidneys have one characteristic different from all the other inner depots, that is, the kidneys have two (segments). The left one is the kidney; the right one is the gate of life. The kidney is responsible for the yin (qi); the gate of life is responsible for the yang (qi). Hence the kidneys are also called "depot of water and fire."

6. 胆：胆为清净之腑，主决断。胆与肝为表里，肝气虽强，非胆不断，肝胆相济，勇敢乃成。人身心为"君火"，胆与命门为"相火"，胆火偏亢，则出现急躁易怒，头胀，胸闷，胁痛，口苦，呕吐苦水等症。

7. 胃：胃为水谷之海，主受纳。胃与脾为表里，前人虽分胃司受纳，脾司消化，但胃的基本功能既能受纳，亦能消化，故脾胃往往相提并论。并认为不能受纳，也就谈不到消化。

Transliteration 4.5

6. Dǎn: dǎn wéi qīng-jìng zhī fǔ, zhǔ jué-duàn. Dǎn yǔ gān wéi biǎo lǐ, gān-qì suī qiáng, fēi dǎn bù duàn, gān dǎn xiāng jì, yǒng-gǎn nǎi chéng. Rén-shēn xīn wéi "jūn-huǒ," dǎn yǔ mìng-mén wéi "xiāng-huǒ," dǎn-huǒ piān-kàng, zé chū-xiàn jí-zào yì-nù, tóu-zhàng, xiōng-mèn, xié-tòng, kǒu-kǔ, ǒu-tù kǔ shuǐ děng zhèng.

7. Wèi: wèi wéi shuǐ-gǔ zhī hǎi, zhǔ shòu-nà. Wèi yǔ pí wéi biǎo lǐ, qián-rén suī fēn wèi sī shòu-nà, pí sī xiāo-huà, dàn wèi de jī-běn gōng-néng jì néng shòu-nà, yì néng xiāo-huà, gù pí wèi wǎng-wǎng xiāng-tí bìng-lùn. Bìng rèn-wéi bù néng shòu-nà, yě jiù tán-bù-dào xiāo-huà.

Vocabulary 4.5

清净	qīng-jìng	purity
决断	jué-duàn	decide
虽	suī	even though
非 ... 不 ...	fēi ... bù ...	only if ... is ...
济	jì	assist
勇敢	yǒng-gǎn	courage
人身	rén-shēn	human body
君火	jūn-huǒ	ruler fire
相火	xiāng-huǒ	minister fire
胆火	dǎn-huǒ	fire of the gallbladder
偏亢	piān-kàng	unilaterally excessive
急躁	jí-zào	rashness and impatience
易怒	yì-nù	tendency to become angry
胸闷	xiōng-mèn	chest pressure
胁痛	xié-tòng	pain in the ribs
口苦	kǒu-kǔ	bitter feeling in the mouth
呕吐	ǒu-tù	vomiting
海	hǎi	sea
受纳	shòu-nà	intake

相提并论	xiāng-tí bìng-lùn	refer to (various things) together
谈不到	tán-bù-dào	cannot be said; be impossible

Translation 4.5

6. The gallbladder: The gallbladder is the palace of purity; it is responsible for decision making. The gallbladder and the liver form outer and inner. Even though the liver qi may be strong, (the liver) will not be able to pass any decisions without the gallbladder. If liver and gallbladder assist each other, courage forms. In the human body, the heart represents the "ruler fire," while the gallbladder together with the gate of life represent the "minister fire." If the fire of the gallbladder is unilaterally excessive, pathoconditions such as restlessness and a tendency toward anger, head ache, and chest pressure, pain in the ribs, a bitter feeling in the mouth, and vomiting of bitter liquid appear.

7. The stomach: The stomach is the sea of water and grain; it is responsible for intake. The stomach and the spleen form outer and inner. In ancient times, the people differentiated (in that they declared) the stomach regulates the intake, and the spleen regulates the digestion (of food), but it is the basic functions of the stomach that enable an intake (of food), and that enable digestion. Hence stomach and spleen are often referred to together. (The people in former times) held the opinion that (if the stomach) is unable to take in, no digestion is possible either.

8. 小肠：小肠为受盛之腑，主化物。小肠承受胃中腐熟的水谷，进一步分别清浊，使精华归于五脏贮藏，糟粕归于六腑排泄，并将糟粕中的水液归于膀胱，渣滓归于大肠。这些都是小肠化物的工作。

9. 大肠：大肠为传导之府，主排泄。大肠接受小肠糟粕，负责输送排泄，为整个消化过程的最后阶段。由于大肠的功能是传导糟粕，职司大便，故凡大便闭结，或泄泻，以及痢疾和便血等，都从大肠着手，而有通导，润泽，固涩等不同的疗法。

Transliteration 4.6

8. Xiǎo-cháng: xiǎo-cháng wéi shòu shèng zhī fǔ, zhǔ huà wù. Xiǎo-cháng chéng-shòu wèi zhōng fǔ-shú de shuǐ-gǔ, jìn-yī-bù fēn-bié qīng zhuó, shǐ jīng-huá guī-yú wǔ-zàng zhù-cáng, zāo-pò guī-yú liù-fǔ pái-xiè, bìng jiāng zāo-pò zhōng de shuǐ-yè guī-yú páng-guāng, zhā-zǐ guī-yú dà-cháng. Zhè-xiē dōu-shì xiǎo-cháng huà wù de gōng-zuò.

9. Dà-cháng: dà-cháng wéi chuán-dǎo zhī fǔ, zhǔ pái-xiè. Dà-cháng jiē-shòu xiǎo-cháng zāo-pò, fù-zé shū-sòng pái-xiè, wéi zhěng-gè xiāo-huà guò-chéng de zuì-hòu jiē-duàn. Yóu-yú dà-cháng de gōng-néng shì chuán-dǎo zāo-pò, zhí-sī dà-biàn, gù fán dà-biàn bì-jié, huò xiè-xiè, yǐ jí lì-ji hé biàn-xuè děng, dōu cóng dà-cháng zhuó-shǒu, ér yǒu tōng-dǎo, rùn-zé, gù-sè děng bù-tóng de liáo-fǎ.

Vocabulary 4.6

承受	chéng-shòu	take in; receive
腐熟	fǔ-shú	decompose
进一步	jìn-yī-bù	in a next step; then
浊	zhuó	turbid
归于	guī-yú	turn to
糟粕	zāo-pò	waste
排泄	pái-xiè	excrete
水液	shuǐ-yè	liquid
渣滓	zhā-zǐ	solid dregs
府	fǔ	palace

接受	jiē-shòu	receive
负责	fù-zé	be responsible for (something)
输送	shū-sòng	transportation
整个	zhěng-gè	entire
最后	zuì-hòu	very last
阶段	jiē-duàn	phase
职司	zhí-sī	regulate; manage
闭结	bì-jié	constipation
痢疾	lì-ji	diarrhea
便血	biàn-xuè	blood-stools
着手	zhuó-shǒu	treat
通导	tōng-dǎo	purge
润泽	rùn-zé	moisten
固涩	gù-sè	contract; (application of) astringent (remedies)
疗法	liáo-fǎ	therapeutic method
等	... děng	... and so on; such as ...

Translation 4.6

8. The small intestine: The small intestine is the palace of receiving abundance; it is responsible for transforming things. The small intestine takes in the liquid and the solid food that have been decomposed in the stomach. Then it separates the clear from the turbid, and causes the essence to turn to the five depots for storage, and the waste to turn to the six palaces for excretion. In addition it makes the liquids in the waste turn to the bladder, and the solid dregs turn to the large intestine. All these are functions of the small intestine (associated with its) transformation of things.

9. The large intestine: The large intestine is the palace of transmission; it is responsible for excretion. The large intestine receives the waste from the small intestine, and it is in charge of (its further) transportation and excretion. It represents the very last phase in the entire process of

digestion. Because the functions of the large intestine include the conveyance of waste, and the management of stools, (pathoconditions) such as constipation, diarrhea, as well as diuretic illnesses and blood-stools are all dealt with starting from the large intestine. (For this purpose) different therapeutic methods exist, such as purging, moistening, or (the application of) astringent (remedies).

10. 膀胱：膀胱为州都之官，司气化。膀胱为水液潴汇之处，气化不利，则小便癃闭；气化不约，则遗溺，小便不禁。但膀胱的气化与肾有关系，肾气足则能化，肾气虚则不能化，故治小便不利或不禁，有时应用温肾之法。

11. 三焦：三焦为决渎之官，主行水。三焦由上焦，中焦，下焦三部分组成。它的主要作用为疏通水道，例如治停水胀满，常用利气来帮助行水，所谓利气，多用疏畅三焦的药物。

Transliteration 4.7

10. Páng-guāng: páng-guāng wéi zhōu-dū zhī guān, sī qì-huà. Páng-guāng wéi shuǐ-yè zhū-huì zhī chù, qì-huà bù-lì, zé xiǎo-biàn-lóng-bì; qì-huà bù-yuē, zé yí-niào, xiǎo-biàn bù-jīn. Dàn páng-guāng de qì-huà yǔ shèn yǒu guān-xi, shèn-qì zú zé néng huà, shèn-qì xū zé bù néng huà, gù zhì xiǎo-biàn bù-lì huò bù-jīn, yǒu-shí yīng yòng wēn shèn zhī fǎ.

11. Sān-jiāo: sān-jiāo wéi jué dú zhī guān, zhǔ xíng shuǐ. Sān-jiāo yóu shàng-jiāo, zhōng-jiāo, xià-jiāo sān bù-fèn zǔ-chéng. Tā-de zhǔ-yào zuò-yòng wéi shū-tōng shuǐ-dào, lì-rú zhì tíng-shuǐ zhàng-mǎn, cháng yòng lì-qì lái bāng-zhù xíng shuǐ, suǒ-wèi lì-qì, duō yòng shū-chàng sān-jiāo de yào-wù.

Vocabulary 4.7

州都	zhōu-dū	"Regional Rectifier" (ancient offical title)
官	guān	official
气化	qì-huà	qi transformation
潴汇	zhū-huì	gather water
不利	bù-lì	impeded flow; blockage of a passage
小便	xiǎo-biàn	urine
小便癃闭	xiǎo-biàn-lóng-bì	retention of urine
不约	bù-yuē	unrestrained
遗溺	yí-niào	enuresis
不禁	bù-jīn	uncontrolled
肾气	shèn-qì	kidney qi
足	zú	sufficient
决	jué	open; clear
渎	dú	ditch
行	xíng	make move; transmit
中焦	zhōng-jiāo	central burner

疏通	shū-tōng	dredge; make passable
水道	shuǐ-dào	water way
停水	tíng-shuǐ	stagnant water
胀满	zhàng-mǎn	swelling and fullness
利气	lì-qì	stimulate the qi (flow)
帮助	bāng-zhù	assist
疏畅	shū-chàng	open; make passable

Translation 4.7

10. The bladder: The bladder is the official (carrying the title) "Regional Rectifier;" it is in charge of the transformation of qi.[1] The bladder is the place where the liquids gather; if the transformation of the qi is impeded, then the urine will be retained. If the transformation of qi is unrestricted, then there will be bed-wetting and restrained flow of urine. However, the qi transformation of the bladder is related to the (condition of the) kidneys. If the qi of the kidneys is sufficient, then (the bladder) is able to transform (qi); if the qi of the kidneys is depleted, then (the bladder) cannot transform (any qi). Hence to treat impeded or unrestrained (flow of urine), it is sometimes advisable to employ (therapeutic) methods to warm the kidneys.

11. The triple burner: The triple burner is the official for clearing the ditches; it is responsible for transmitting water. The triple burner consists of upper burner, central burner, and lower burner. Its major function is to dredge the water ways. For example, to treat swelling and fullness (resulting from) stagnating water, (we) often use (the technique of) stimulating the flow of qi to assist (the triple burner) in transmitting the water. For this so-called stimulation of the flow of qi (we) often use drugs that open the triple burner.

Note

1 The designation of the bladder with the ancient offical title "Regional Rectifier" (responsible for identifying and classifying all males considered qualified for government service) is documented first in the association of all the so-called "depots" and "palaces" constituting the human organism with central positions in the hierarchy of officials governing the social organism in the *Huang Di Nei-jing su-wen* 黄帝内经素问, ch. 3, treatise 8.

Text 4.8

脏腑之外尚有奇恒之府，即脑，髓，骨，脉，胆，女子胞。奇恒的意义是似脏非脏，似腑非腑，形虽似腑而作用似脏；是异乎寻常的一种内脏。它们在人体中也是极其重要的部分。这些奇恒之府并不是孤立的，和脏腑都有联系，比如脑和心，肝有关系，又因脑和髓有关，髓又和骨有关，骨属于肾，脑又和肾有关；女子胞即子宫属肝，由于行经，养胎等与血有关，故又和心，脾有关了。与奇恒之府对称的还有传化之府，即胃，大肠，小肠，三焦，膀胱，这五个腑，在六腑中都是属于消化系统。如上所述，全身组织都是有机的联系，是完整的不可分离的。

Transliteration 4.8

Zàng-fǔ zhī-wài shàng yǒu qí-héng zhī fǔ, jí nǎo, suǐ, gǔ, mài, dǎn, nǚ-zǐ-bāo. Qí-héng de yì-yì shì sì zàng fēi zàng, sì fǔ fēi fǔ, xíng suī sì fǔ ér zuò-yòng sì zàng; shì yì-hū-xún-cháng de yī zhǒng nèi-zàng. Tā-men zài rén-tǐ zhōng yě shì jí-qí zhòng-yào de bù-fèn. Zhè-xiē qí-héng zhī fǔ bìng bù shì gū-lì de, hé zàng-fǔ dōu yǒu lián-xì, bǐ-rú nǎo hé xīn, gān yǒu guān-xi, yòu yīn nǎo hé suǐ yǒu-guān, suǐ yòu hé gǔ yǒu-guān, gǔ shǔ-yú shèn, nǎo yòu hé shèn yǒu-guān; nǚ-zǐ-bāo jí zǐ-gōng shǔ gān, yóu-yú xíng-jīng, yǎng tāi děng yǔ xuè yǒu-guān, gù yòu hé xīn, pí yǒu-guān le. Yǔ qí-héng zhī fǔ duì-chèn de hái-yǒu chuán-huà zhī fǔ, jí wèi, dà-cháng, xiǎo-cháng, sān-jiāo, páng-guāng, zhè wǔ gè fǔ, zài liù fǔ zhōng dōu-shì shǔ-yú xiāo-huà xì-tǒng. Rú shàng-suǒ-shù, quán-shēn zǔ-zhī dōu-shì yǒu-jī de lián-xì, shì wán-zhěng de bù-kě fèn-lí de.

Vocabulary 4.8

之外	zhī-wài	in addition to
奇恒	qí-héng	extraordinary
脑	nǎo	brain
髓	suǐ	marrow

女子胞	nǚ-zǐ-bāo	womb; uterus
似	sì	appear like
非	fēi	be not
形	xíng	shape
异乎寻常	yì-hū-xún-cháng	unusual
并	bìng	(particle emphasizing the following negation)
有关	yǒu-guān	be related to
行经	xíng-jīng	menstruation
养	yǎng	nourish
胎	tāi	fetus
对称	duì-chèn	symmetrical
系统	xì-tǒng	system
上所述	shàng-suǒ-shù	said above
完整	wán-zhěng	integrated
不可	bù-kě	cannot
分离	fēn-lí	separate

Translation 4.8

In addition to the depots and palaces, there are also extraordinary palaces, namely, the brain, the marrow, the bones, the vessels, the gallbladder[1] and the womb. The meaning of "extraordinary" is that (these palaces) appear like depots but are not depots; they appear like palaces but are not palaces. Even though their physical shape resembles (that of the) palaces, their functions resemble (those of the) depots. They are a type of unusual inner depots. They too are very important parts of the human body. These extraordinary palaces are by no means isolated; they are related to all the depots and palaces. For example, the brain is related to the heart and to the liver; also, because the brain is related to the marrow, and (because) furthermore the marrow is related to the bones, and (because) the bones belong to the kidneys, the brain is also related to the kidneys. The womb is the uterus, and is related to the liver. Because mentruation and the nourishment of the fetus are related to the blood, the (uterus) is also related to the heart and to the spleen. In symmetry to the extraordinary palaces are the palaces of transmission and transformation; namely, the stomach, the large intestine, the small intestine, the triple burner, and the bladder. Among the six palaces, these five palaces all belong to the digestive system. As was said above, all organic relationships of the structure of the entire body are integrated, and cannot be separated.

Note

1 This association of the gallbladder with the "extraordinary palaces" is documented in the *Huang Di Nei-jing su-wen*, ch. 3, treatise 11. Because the gallbladder is usually counted among the regular "palaces," most commentators of the *Huang Di Nei-jing su-wen* consider the present passage as an error previously introduced into the text in pre-Tang times.

Text 5.1

气和血并重，更把气作为血的统帅，这是中医生理上的一种认识方法。气的名称相当多，有元气，真气，精气，这些都是指整个人体内气血和其它物质及能力，名虽异而实为一种。另有阳气，阴气之称，这是从元气内分别两大作用，说明一种能保卫体表，另一种能保持精力不使亏耗，故也叫真阳，真阴。还有宗气，中气，是指元气中有一部分属于上焦肺，另一部分属于中焦脾胃，所以亦叫肺气，胃气。概括的说，均为元气。

Transliteration 5.1

Qì hé xuè bìng zhòng, gèng bǎ qì zuò-wéi xuè de tǒng-shuài, zhè shì zhōng-yī shēng-lǐ shàng de yī zhǒng rèn-shi fāng-fǎ. Qì de míng-chēng xiāng-dāng duō, yǒu yuán-qì, zhēn-qì, jīng-qì, zhè-xiē dōu-shì zhǐ zhěng-gè rén-tǐ nèi qì xuè hé qí-tā wù-zhì jí néng-lì, míng suī yì ér shí wéi yī zhǒng. Lìng-yǒu yáng-qì, yīn-qì zhī chēng, zhè shì cóng yuán-qì nèi fēn-bié liǎng dà zuò-yòng, shuō-míng yī zhǒng néng bǎo-wèi tǐ-biǎo, lìng-yī zhǒng néng bǎo-chí jīng-lì bù shǐ kuī-hào, gù yě jiào zhēn-yáng, zhēn-yīn. Hái-yǒu zōng-qì, zhōng-qì, shì zhǐ yuán-qì zhōng yǒu yī bù-fèn shǔ-yú shàng-jiāo fèi, lìng-yī bù-fèn shǔ-yú zhōng-jiāo pí wèi, suǒ-yǐ yì jiào fèi-qì, wèi-qì. Gài-kuò-de-shuō, jūn wéi yuán-qì.

Vocabulary 5.1

统帅	tǒng-shuài	commander
认识	rèn-shi	recognize; cognition
名称	míng-chēng	designation; name
相当	xiāng-dāng	quite
元气	yuán-qì	original qi
真气	zhēn-qì	true qi
名	míng	name
异	yì	be different
另有	lìng-yǒu	in addition there is/are
阳气	yáng-qì	yang qi
从 ... 内	cóng ... nèi	from within
大	dà	big; major

另一	lìng-yī	another
精力	jīng-lì	vigor
亏耗	kuī-hào	consumed; worn away; depleted; lost
真阳	zhēn-yáng	true yang (qi)
真阴	zhēn-yīn	true yin (qi)
宗气	zōng-qì	ancestral qi
中气	zhōng-qì	central qi
胃气	wèi-qì	stomach qi

Translation 5.1

Qi and blood are equally important. Furthermore, it is a cognitive convention in the physiology of Chinese medicine to consider qi to be the commander of the blood. The designations of qi are quite numerous – there are (such names as) original qi, true qi, and essential qi – (and) all these (designations) serve to refer to the qi and to the blood, as well as to any other substances or abilities within the entire human body. Even though they are different in name, they are in fact identical. In addition, there are the designations yang qi and yin qi. That is, within the original qi two major functions are distinguished to explain that one type (of qi) is capable of protecting the body's exterior, and that another type (of qi) is capable of conserving (the body's vigor) and of preventing its loss. Hence (these two types of qi) are also called true yang (qi), and true yin (qi). There are, furthermore, the (designations) ancestral qi[1] and central qi. They refer (to the fact that) within the original influences there is one part that belongs to the upper warmer and to the lung, and another part that belongs to the central warmer, and to spleen and stomach. Consequently, (these two types of qi) are also called lung qi and stomach qi. Generally speaking, they all represent original qi.

Note

1 The etymology of the term "ancestral qi" may have originated in a notion of an original qi received from the ancestors. This type of qi is focussed in the chest, hence it is often translated as "pectoral qi" in modern Chinese dictionaries.

气血的气，有些地方代表能力，有些地方代表物质，因而有气属无形，血为有形的说法。我们的体会，前人把气和血对待提出，血是物质，气也应该是物质，气所发生的作用就是"能力"。血液循行脉内全身受其营养，气能改善血液的功能和帮助血液的正常运行，二者是构成人体正常生理活动的重要因素，而是绝对不能分离的。假使气受到心理上，环境上的刺激，无论情志方面的喜，怒，哀，乐，气候方面的冷，热，以及工作方面的劳逸，都会影响到血。因此，前人特别重视气，称作"气为血帅"，又说"百病皆生于气"。

Transliteration 5.2

Qì xuè de qì, yǒu-xiē dì-fāng dài-biǎo néng-lì, yǒu-xiē dì-fāng dài-biǎo wù-zhì, yīn-ér yǒu qì shǔ wú-xíng, xuè wéi yǒu-xíng de shuō-fǎ. Wǒ-men-de tǐ-huì, qián-rén bǎ qì hé xuè duì-dài tí-chū, xuè shì wù-zhì, qì yě yīng-gāi shì wù-zhì, qì suǒ fā-shēng de zuò-yòng jiù-shì "néng-lì." Xuè-yè xún-xíng mài nèi quán-shēn shòu qí yíng-yǎng, qì néng gǎi-shàn xuè-yè de gōng-néng hé bāng-zhù xuè-yè de zhèng-cháng yùn-xíng, èr-zhě shì gòu-chéng rén-tǐ zhèng-cháng shēng-lǐ huó-dòng de zhòng-yào yīn-sù, ér shì jué-duì bù néng fēn-lí de. Jiǎ-shǐ qì shòu-dào xīn-lǐ-shàng, huán-jìng shàng de cì-jī, wú-lùn qíng-zhì fāng-miàn de xǐ, nù, āi, lè, qì-hòu fāng-miàn de lěng, rè, yǐ-jí gōng-zuò fāng-miàn de láo yì, dōu huì yǐng-xiǎng dào xuè. Yīn-cǐ, qián-rén tè-bié zhòng-shì qì, chēng-zuò "qì wéi xuè shuài," yòu shuō "bǎi bìng jiē shēng yú qì."

Vocabulary 5.2

些	xiē	some
有些	yǒu-xiē	there are some; some
地方	dì-fāng	location, place
无形	wú-xíng	formless
有形	yǒu-xíng	tangible
说法	shuō-fǎ	opinion; statement

我们的	wǒ-men-de	our
体会	tǐ-huì	understand (by personal experience rather than rationally); understanding
对待	duì-dài	treat
提出	tí-chū	propose
改善	gǎi-shàn	improve
二者	èr-zhě	both
因素	yīn-sù	element; factor
绝对	jué-duì	definitely
假使	jiǎ-shǐ	if; when
心理上	xīn-lǐ-shàng	psychological
环境	huán-jìng	environment
哀	āi	grief
乐	lè	joy
劳	láo	fatigue
逸	yì	idleness
特别	tè-bié	particular; special
帅	shuài	commander
百	bǎi	hundred
皆	jiē	all

Translation 5.2

The qi of the expression "qi and blood" sometimes stands for a power, and sometimes for a substance. Hence there is one opinion (stating) qi belongs to the formless, the blood is tangible. According to our understanding, people of former times proposed to treat qi and blood (as follows): the blood is a substance, and qi should also be a substance. The effect brought forth by the qi, though, is a "power." The blood moves inside the vessels, and the entire body receives its nourishment (through the blood). Qi is able to improve the ability of the blood, and to assist the normal movement of the blood. The two constitute important elements in the generation of the normal physiological activities of the human body, and they are definitely inseparable. When qi receives psychological or environmental stimuli no matter whether (they originate from) the realm of minds, (such as) happiness, anger, grief, or joy, (or from) the realm of work, (such as) fatigue or idleness they all can exert an influence on the blood. Hence people of former times paid particular attention to qi, stating "qi is the commander of the blood," or "all illnesses emerge from qi."

Text 5.3

一般的说，血分病虽当用血分药治疗，但还有理气和血，行气逐瘀，血脱益气等治法，这是因为气行则血行，气滞则血滞，要使血液循行正常，先使气机舒畅；要使瘀血排除，先使气分通利。在出血不止的症候，还能用补气药来帮助收摄；严重的贫血症，根据阳生则阴长的道理，同样需要用补气药来加速恢复。这些方法，在临症上都是很有效的。中医临症时所称的气，多数是指脏腑机能的障碍，或消化不良等产生的气体。常见的如胸膈痞闷，用气滞，气壅，气郁，气积等名词，作为病理的解释。发生这些症状的病症，也就多用气字为病名，如气膈，气臌，气淋和肝气，胃气痛等等。

Transliteration 5.3

Yī-bān-de-shuō, xuè-fèn-bìng suī dāng yòng xuè-fèn-yào zhì-liáo, dàn hái-yǒu lǐ-qì hé xuè, xíng-qì zhú-yū, xuè-tuō yì-qì děng zhì-fǎ, zhè shì yīn-wèi qì xíng zé xuè xíng, qì zhì zé xuè zhì, yào shǐ xuè-yè xún-xíng zhèng-cháng, xiān shǐ qì-jī shū-chàng; yào shǐ yū-xuè pái-chú, xiān shǐ qì-fèn tōng-lì. Zài chū-xuè-bù-zhǐ de zhèng-hòu, hái néng yòng bǔ-qì-yào lái bāng-zhù shōu-shè; yán-zhòng de pín-xuè zhèng, gēn-jù yáng shēng zé yīn zhǎng de dào-lǐ, tóng-yàng xū-yào yòng bǔ-qì-yào lái jiā-sù huī-fù. Zhè-xiē fāng-fǎ, zài lín-zhèng shàng dōu-shì hěn yǒu-xiào de. Zhōng-yī lín-zhèng shí suǒ chēng de qì, duō-shù shì zhǐ zàng-fǔ jī-néng de zhàng-ài, huò xiāo-huà bù liáng děng chǎn-shēng de qì-tǐ. Cháng-jiàn de rú xiōng gé pǐ-mèn, yòng qì-zhì, qì-yōng, qì-yù, qì-jī děng míng-cí, zuò-wéi bìng-lǐ de jiě-shì. Fā-shēng zhè-xiē zhèng-zhuàng de bìng-zhèng, yě jiù duō yòng qì zì wéi bìng-míng, rú qì-gé, qì-gǔ, qì-lín hé gān-qì, wèi-qì tòng děng-děng.

Vocabulary 5.3

分	fèn	section
血分病	xuè-fèn-bìng	illnesses in the section of the blood; blood illnesses
血分药	xuè-fèn-yào	drugs active in the section of the blood
行气	xíng-qì	make qi move
逐	zhú	eliminate; expel
瘀	yū	stagnate; stagnation
逐瘀	zhú-yū	expel stagnations
血脱	xuè-tuō	blood loss
益	yì	increase
益气	yì-qì	increase qi
因为	yīn-wèi	because
滞	zhì	sluggish
先	xiān	first
气机	qì-jī	qi movement
瘀血	yū-xuè	stagnant blood
排除	pái-chú	eliminate
气分	qì-fèn	qi section
通利	tōng-lì	open for passage
出血不止	chū-xuè-bù-zhǐ	incessant bleeding
需要	xū-yào	must; needs to
还	hái	also; in addition
补气药	bǔ-qì-yào	drug supplementing qi
收摄	shōu-shè	acquire
严重	yán-zhòng	serious
加速	jiā-sù	accelerate; speed up
恢复	huī-fù	recovery
很	hěn	very
有效	yǒu-xiào	effective
时	shí	while; during
多数	duō-shù	mostly; often
障碍	zhàng-ài	obstruction

良	liáng	good
产生	chǎn-shēng	produce
气体	qì-tǐ	gas
常见	cháng-jiàn	often
胸	xiōng	chest
膈	gé	diaphragm
痞闷	pǐ-mèn	blocks and chest pressure
气滞	qì-zhì	qi sluggishness
气壅	qì-yōng	qi obstruction
气郁	qì-yù	qi stagnation
字	zì	character of Chinese script
病名	bìng-míng	illness name
气膈	qì-gé	qi blockage
气臌	qì-gǔ	qi bloating
气淋	qì-lín	qi strangury

Translation 5.3

Generally speaking, even though illnesses in the section of blood must be treated with drugs for the section of blood, there are also therapeutic patterns (aiming at) regulating qi to harmonize the blood, moving qi to expel stagnations (of blood), or to increase qi in case of blood loss. The reason is, when the qi moves, the blood moves; when the qi is sluggish, the blood is sluggish. If it is intended to let the blood move normally, it should be seen to it first that the qi flow is unimpeded. If it is intended to eliminate stagnant blood, the qi section should first be opened for passage. In case of pathoconditions of incessant bleeding, drugs supplementing the qi to assist (the body) to acquire (new blood) may be used too. And in case of serious anemia, drugs supplementing the qi to speed up recovery must likewise be employed, according to the principle "when the yang is alive, then the yin grows." All these procedures are very effective in clinical practice.

The (term) qi that is mentioned in clinical situations of Chinese medicine, often refers to gases produced, for instance, by obstructions of the functions of the depots and palaces, or bad digestion. For often seen (conditions) such as (feelings of) block and pressure in the chest and at the diaphragm, (Chinese medicine) employs terms such as qi sluggishness, qi obstruction, qi stagnation, or qi accumulation as pathological explanations. To name the illnesses that give rise to such conditions, (Chinese medicine) also frequently uses the character qi, as for example (in designations such as) qi blockage, qi bloating, or qi dripping, as well as liver qi or stomach qi pain.

Text 5.4

全身都靠血液营养。凡是心脏衰弱或血亏，循行失调，会出现心悸，惊惕，脉来歇止。血液得寒则凝滞，得热则妄行，这寒和热包括外界的寒邪和热邪，饮食的寒凉和辛热，以及体质的偏寒，偏热和肝火偏旺等。故血病主要分为瘀血和出血，当然与气也有密切关系。血虚多起于疲劳过度，创伤出血过多和病后及妇人产后，当已经成为血虚症时，就须从心，肝，脾三脏治疗，必要时并应进一步从肾脏治疗。

Transliteration 5.4

Quán-shēn dōu kào xuè-yè yíng-yǎng. Fán-shì xīn-zàng shuāi-ruò huò xuè-kuī, xún-xíng shī-tiáo, huì chū-xiàn xīn-jì, jīng-tì, mài-lái-xiē-zhǐ. Xuè-yè dé hán zé níng-zhì, dé rè zé wàng xíng, zhè hán hé rè bāo-kuò wài-jiè de hán-xié hé rè-xié, yǐn-shí de hán-liáng hé xīn-rè, yǐ-jí tǐ-zhì de piān hán, piān rè hé gān-huǒ piān wàng děng. Gù xuè-bìng zhǔ-yào fēn-wéi yū-xuè hé chū-xuè, dāng-rán yǔ qì yě yǒu mì-qiè guān-xi. Xuè-xū duō qǐ yú pí-láo guò-dù, chuāng-shāng chū-xuè guò-duō hé bìng hòu jí fù-rén chǎn hòu, dāng yǐ-jīng chéng-wéi xuè-xū zhèng shí, jiù xū cóng xīn, gān, pí sān zàng zhì-liáo, bì-yào shí bìng yīng jìn-yī-bù cóng shèn-zàng zhì-liáo.

Vocabulary 5.4

靠	kào	depend on
血亏	xuè-kuī	anemia
失调	shī-tiáo	lose rhythm
脉来歇止	mài-lái-xiē-zhǐ	breaks in the arrival of the pulse
得	dé	receive
凝滞	níng-zhì	congeal and stagnate
妄	wàng	erratic
外界	wài-jiè	external world; environment
寒邪	hán-xié	cold evil
热邪	rè-xié	heat evil
饮食	yǐn-shí	drink and food
寒凉	hán-liáng	cold
体质	tǐ-zhì	physical constitution
偏	piān	one-sided
旺	wàng	effulgent
血病	xuè-bìng	blood illness
出血	chū-xuè	hemorrhage
当然	dāng-rán	of course
疲劳	pí-láo	fatigue

过度	guò-dù	excessive
创伤	chuāng-shāng	wound
过多	guò-duō	too much
妇人	fù-rén	woman
产	chǎn	deliver; delivery
须	xū	must

Translation 5.4

The entire body depends on the nourishment (provided by) the blood. Whenever the heart is weak, or in case of anemia, when (as a result) the movement (of the blood) loses its proper rhythm, this may produce (conditions such as) palpitation, fright, or breaks in the arrival of the pulse. When the blood receives cold, then it will congeal and slacken. When it receives heat, then it will move erratically. This cold and heat (just referred to) include the cold evil and the heat evil of the external world, the coldness and the acrid heat of drink and food, and any unbalanced cold, unbalanced heat, and effulgence of the liver fire as far as the physical constitution is concerned. Hence blood illnesses are divided mainly into (those of) hemostasis and hemorrhage, and they are, of course, closely related to the (condition of the) qi. Blood depletion often emerges from excessive fatigue, and from excessive bleeding from wounds, as well as following illness or, in females, after delivery. When a condition of blood depletion has already developed, it is treated through the three depots heart, liver, and spleen. If necessary, it should, furthermore, be treated through the kidneys.

Text 5.5

精是人体生长，发育以及生殖能力的物质基础。中医把精归于肾脏，精为生命的基础。所以称肾为"先天"。待到出生以后，便靠饮食来给养，这是脾胃的作用，故称脾胃为"后天"，并在临症上认为先天不足，可用后天来调养。精，对于体力有密切影响，故患有遗精的人，多呈腰酸，背痛，腿弱。由于肾主藏精，一般对上述症状称之为肾亏，以补肾为主。必须指出，中医书上有很多地方是指广义的精，就是指人体的精气。不能和狭义的精混为一谈。

Transliteration 5.5

Jīng shì rén-tǐ shēng-zhǎng, fā-yù yǐ-jí shēng-zhí néng-lì de wù-zhì jī-chǔ. Zhōng-yī bǎ jīng guī-yú shèn-zàng, jīng wéi shēng-mìng de jī-chǔ. Suǒ-yǐ chēng shèn wéi "xiān-tiān." Dài-dào chū-shēng yǐ-hòu, biàn kào yǐn-shí lái jǐ-yǎng, zhè shì pí wèi de zuò-yòng, gù chēng pí wèi wéi "hòu-tiān," bìng zài lín-zhèng shàng rèn-wéi xiān-tiān bù-zú, kě yòng hòu-tiān lái tiáo-yǎng. Jīng, duì-yú tǐ-lì yǒu mì-qiè yǐng-xiǎng, gù huàn yǒu yí-jīng de rén, duō chéng yāo-suān, bèi-tòng, tuǐ ruò. Yóu-yú shèn zhǔ cáng jīng, yī-bān duì shàng-shù zhèng-zhuàng chēng zhī wéi shèn-kuī, yǐ bǔ shèn wéi zhǔ. Bì-xū zhǐ-chū, zhōng-yī shū shàng yǒu hěn duō dì-fāng shì zhǐ guǎng-yì de jīng, jiù-shì zhǐ rén-tǐ de jīng-qì. Bù néng hé xiá-yì de jīng hùn-wéi-yī-tán.

Vocabulary 5.5

生长	shēng-zhǎng	growth
发育	fā-yù	development
基础	jī-chǔ	basis
归于	guī-yú	associate with
待	dài	wait
... 以后	... yǐ-hòu	after ...
待到 ... 以后	dài-dào ... yǐ-hòu	after ...
出生	chū-shēng	be born; give birth
给养	jǐ-yǎng	nourishment
调养	tiáo-yǎng	regulate nourishment
体力	tǐ-lì	physical strength
患	huàn	suffer (from an illness)

呈	chéng	manifest; present
腰酸	yāo-suān	lumbar pain
背痛	bèi-tòng	back pain
腿	tuǐ	leg
肾亏	shèn-kuī	kidney deficiency
书	shū	text
广义	guǎng-yì	broad sense
狭义	xiá-yì	narrow sense
混为一谈	hùn-wéi-yī-tán	speak of separate entities as a single entity; confuse

Translation 5.5

Essence is the material basis of the growth, development, and reproductive power of the human body. Chinese medicine associates essence with the kidneys; essence is the basis of life. Hence (Chinese medicine) calls the kidneys the "earlier dependences." Once (the human body) is born, it depends on food and beverages for the provision of nourishment. This is the function of spleen and stomach. Hence (Chinese medicine) calls spleen and stomach the "later dependences." Also, in clinical practice, (Chinese medicine) thinks that if the (supply offered by the) earlier dependences is insufficient, the later dependences can be used to regulate the nourishment. Essence has a close influence on (a person's) physical strength. Hence persons suffering from (involuntary) seminal efflux often present themselves with lumbar pain, or weakness in their legs. Because the kidneys are responsible for storing essence, the above-mentioned pathoconditions are generally called kidney deficiency, and to supplement the kidneys is considered of primary importance (here). It should be emphasized that the many places in Chinese medical texts that refer to essence in a broad sense do in fact refer to the essential qi of the human body. (These references, though,) must not be confused with essence in a narrow sense.

Text 5.6

前人认为人体的各组织都是有形的，还有一个高级的，无形的一种能力在主持活动，称它为"神"。假使神能充旺，内脏和形体就活泼，神一涣散，一切不起作用了。神发生病变，便会产生胸膈烦闷，两胁不舒，精神不能自主，手足无力，狂妄不识人，记忆力衰退，前阴萎缩，腰背酸痛不能俯仰转侧等一系列的症状。成方中如朱砂安神丸，琥珀定志丸等，均是治疗这种病的。但是，神不是空洞的，需要物质来营养。这就在治疗神病时候，不能单靠安神定志，必须结合养血，补气等方法了。

Transliteration 5.6

Qián-rén rèn-wéi rén-tǐ de gè zǔ-zhī dōu-shì yǒu-xíng de, hái-yǒu yī ge gāo-jí de, wú-xíng de yī zhǒng néng-lì zài zhǔ-chí huó-dòng, chēng tā wéi "shén." Jiǎ-shǐ shén néng chōng wàng, nèi-zàng hé xíng-tǐ jiù huó-po, shén yī huàn-sàn, yī-qiè bù qǐ zuò-yòng le. Shén fā-shēng bìng-biàn, biàn huì chǎn-shēng xiōng gé fán-mèn, liǎng xié bù-shū, jīng-shén bù néng zì-zhǔ, shǒu zú wú-lì, kuáng-wàng bù shí rén, jì-yì-lì shuāi-tuì, qián yīn wěi-suō, yāo bèi suān tòng bù néng fǔ-yǎng zhuǎn-cè děng yī xì-liè de zhèng-zhuàng. Chéng-fāng zhōng rú zhū-shā ān-shén wán, hǔ-pò dìng-zhì wán děng, jūn shì zhì-liáo zhè zhǒng bìng de. Dàn-shì, shén bù shì kōng-dòng de, xū-yào wù-zhì lái yíng-yǎng. Zhè jiù zài zhì-liáo shén-bìng shí-hòu, bù néng dān kào ān-shén dìng-zhì, bì-xū jié-hé yǎng-xuè, bǔ-qì děng fāng-fǎ le.

Vocabulary 5.6

高级	gāo-jí	high-level
在	zài	(particle indicating the continuous form of the subsequent verb)
主持	zhǔ-chí	direct; be responsible for
充	chōng	complete
活泼	huó-po	active
一	yī	as soon as
涣散	huàn-sàn	slacken
烦闷	fán-mèn	uneasiness and chest pressure

不舒	bù-shū	tense
狂妄	kuáng-wàng	frantic
识	shí	recognize
记忆力	jì-yì-lì	memory
萎缩	wěi-suō	shrink
腰	yāo	lumbus
背	bèi	back
俯仰	fǔ-yǎng	lower or lift (the head)
转侧	zhuǎn-cè	turn to the side
转	zhuàn	turn around
系列	xì-liè	series
成方	chéng-fāng	established prescription
朱砂	zhū-shā	cinnabar
安神	ān-shén	pacify the spirit
丸	wán	pill
琥珀	hǔ-pò	amber
定志	dìng-zhì	stabilize the will
但是	dàn-shì	however; but
空洞	kōng-dòng	empty
这就	zhè-jiù	that is
神病	shén-bìng	spirit illness
时候	shí-hòu	time
在 ... 时候	zài ... shí-hòu	while; during ...
单	dān	only
养血	yǎng-xuè	nourish the blood
补气	bǔ-qì	supplement the qi

Translation 5.6

People of former times thought that all structures of the human body are tangible, and that there is, in addition, a kind of a high-level, shapeless power directing the (body's) activities. They called this "spirit." As long as the faculties of the spirit are complete and vigorous, the internal depots and the physical body are active. As soon as the spirit slackens, none of them will fulfill its functions any longer. When the spirit undergoes pathological changes, these may generate a whole series of conditions, such as a feeling of uneasiness and pressure in the chest and at the diaphragm, tensions in both flanks, inability of the mind to control itself, lack of strength in hands and feet, frantic behavior and failure to recognize people, failing memory, shrinking of the genital organs, soreness and pain in the lumbus and back, and inability to lower or lift the head, or to turn to the side. Among the established prescriptions, the "pills with cinnabar to pacify the spirit" or the "pills with amber to stabilize the will" serve both alike to treat these kinds of illness. However, the spirit is not an empty (idea); it needs substance for nourishment. That is, whenever an illness of the spirit is treated, there must be no exclusive reliance on (patterns to) pacify the spirit, or to stabilize the mind. It is essential to combine (such approaches) with methods to nourish the blood and to supplement qi.

Text 5.7

津和液是两种不同性质的液质，但不等于一般所说的水分。故津液亡脱，在津为腠理开，汗大泄，在液为身体萎枯，毛发憔悴，耳鸣，胫酸，骨属屈伸不利。津液可以转化为血，因而中医有津血同源的说法，理由是亡血有吐，衄，便，尿四大症，亡津亦有呕，吐，消，汗四大症。吐血出于贲门，与呕吐同；鼻衄名为红汗，与汗出同；便血出于大肠，与下利同；尿血出于胞中，与下消同。两者相比，性质相似。故保津即所以保血，养血亦可以生津，临症上常把亡血和亡津液并提。

Transliteration 5.7

Jīn hé yè shì liǎng zhǒng bù-tóng xìng-zhì de yè-zhì, dàn bù děng-yú yī-bān suǒ-shuō-de shuǐ-fèn. Gù jīn-yè wáng-tuō, zài jīn wéi còu-lǐ kāi, hàn dà xiè, zài yè wéi shēn-tǐ wěi-kū, máo-fà qiáo-cuì, ěr-míng, jìng-suān, gǔ shǔ qū shēn bù-lì. Jīn-yè kě-yǐ zhuǎn-huà wéi xuè, yīn-ér zhōng-yī yǒu jīn xuè tóng yuán de shuō-fǎ, lǐ-yóu shì wáng-xuè yǒu tù, nǜ, biàn, niào sì dà zhèng, wáng jīn yì yǒu ǒu, tù, xiāo, hàn sì dà zhèng. Tù-xuè chū-yú bēn-mén, yǔ ǒu-tù tóng; bí-nǜ míng wéi hóng-hàn, yǔ hàn-chū tóng; biàn-xuè chū-yú dà-cháng, yǔ xià-lì tóng; niào-xiě chū-yú bāo zhōng, yǔ xià-xiāo tóng. Liǎng zhě xiāng-bǐ, xìng-zhì xiāng-sì. Gù bǎo jīn jí suǒ-yǐ bǎo xuè, yǎng xuè yì kě-yǐ shēng jīn, lín-zhèng shàng cháng bǎ wáng xuè hé wáng jīn-yè bìng-tí.

Vocabulary 5.7

津	jīn	jin humor
液质	yè-zhì	humors
等于	děng-yú	be comparable to
所说的	suǒ-shuō-de	so-called
水分	shuǐ-fèn	water (fluid) content
津液	jīn-yè	body liquids
亡	wáng	lose; loss
亡脱	wáng-tuō	lose; loss
腠理	còu-lǐ	porous structures
开	kāi	open
泄	xiè	flow off
身体	shēn-tǐ	body

萎枯	wěi-kū	dry up
毛发	máo-fà	hair; body hair
憔悴	qiáo-cuì	wither
屈	qū	bend
伸	shēn	stretch
转化	zhuǎn-huà	transform
同	tóng	common
源	yuán	source
理由	lǐ-yóu	reason; cause
亡血	wáng-xuè	blood loss
衄	nǜ	spontaneous external bleeding
尿	niào	urine
呕	ǒu	vomit; retch
消	xiāo	waste
吐血	tù-xuè	spit blood
出于	chū-yú	leave from
贲门	bēn-mén	lit: "rushing gate;" upper stomach opening
鼻衄	bí-nǜ	nosebleed
红汗	hóng-hàn	"red sweat" (i.e., nosebleed)
汗出	hàn-chū	sweat
下利	xià-lì	diarrhea
尿血	niào-xuè	bloody urine
胞	bāo	bladder
下消	xià-xiāo	downward wasting
相比	xiāng-bǐ	compare
相似	xiāng-sì	be similar
保	bǎo	protect
并提	bìng-tí	refer together

Translation 5.7

Jin humors and ye humors are two liquids of different nature. However, they are not comparable to what is generally called water content. Hence a loss of humors means – in case of jin humors – that the porous structures open and that sweat flows off excessively. In case of ye humors it means that the body dries up, that the hair withers, that the ears ring, that the lower legs ache, and that the bones and joints cannot bend and stretch freely. The humors can transform into blood. Hence Chinese medicine has a saying: "The jin humors and the blood have a common source." The reason is that a loss of blood entails (any of) the four major pathoconditions of vomiting (blood), spontaneous external bleeding, (blood in the) stool, and (blood in the) urine, and that a loss of jin humors equally entails (any of) the four major pathoconditions of vomiting, spitting, wasting, and sweating. Blood that is spat forth leaves (the body) from the upper opening of the stomach. The same applies to vomiting and spitting. Nosebleed is called red sweat; it is identical with sweat leaving (the body). Bloody stool leaves (the body) by way of the large intestine. The same is true of diarrhea. Bloody urine leaves (the body) from the bladder; this is identical with downward wasting.[1] In comparison, the natures of both are similar. Hence to protect the jin humors is (a method) by which the blood is protected too, and to nourish the blood is (a method) by which jin humors are generated too. In clinical practice, a loss of blood and a loss of jin and ye humors are often referred to together.

Note

1 The term xiāo, "wasting," refers to an excessive loss of body liquid through urination. This idea is expressed also in the term used for the illness of xiāo kě, "wasting and thirst," nowadays identified as diabetes, whereby a patient appears to waste away by losing more liquid through urination than is supplemented by quenching a strong thirst.

Text 5.8

津液也能化为汗，涕，泪，涎，唾，主要是属于肾脏，故称肾主五液。脾阳虚弱的人，津液不化，还能凝聚成痰饮，痰饮内阻，津液无以上升，口干不欲饮，当用温药和之。临症上常见的津液缺少症状为口渴，多由热性病引起，常用的生津药，为石斛，麦冬，玉竹，天花粉一类。但轻浅的口渴不一定用生津药，清热则津自回转，生津药性多粘腻，用时应考虑有无流弊。口渴严重的非生津能治，又当进一步与养血，养阴同用。

Transliteration 5.8

Jīn-yè yě néng huà wéi hàn, tì, lèi, xián, tuò, zhǔ-yào shì shǔ-yú shèn-zàng, gù chēng shèn zhǔ wǔ-yè. Pí-yáng xū-ruò de rén, jīn-yè bù huà, hái néng níng-jù chéng tán-yǐn, tán-yǐn nèi zǔ, jīn-yè wú-yǐ shàng-shēng, kǒu gān bù yù yǐn, dāng yòng wēn-yào hé zhī. Lín-zhèng shàng cháng-jiàn de jīn-yè quē-shǎo zhèng-zhuàng wéi kǒu-kě, duō yóu rè-xìng-bìng yǐn-qǐ, cháng-yòng de shēng-jīn-yào, wéi shí-hú, mài-dōng, yù-zhú, tiān-huā-fěn yī lèi. Dàn qīng-qiǎn de kǒu-kě bù yī-dìng yòng shēng-jīn-yào, qīng-rè zé jīn zì huí-zhuǎn, shēng-jīn-yào xìng duō nián-nì, yòng shí yīng kǎo-lǜ yǒu-wú liú-bì. Kǒu-kě yán-zhòng de fēi shēng jīn néng zhì, yòu dāng jìn-yī-bù yǔ yǎng xuè, yǎng yīn tóng yòng.

Vocabulary 5.8

涕	tì	snivel
泪	lèi	tears
涎	xián	saliva
唾	tuò	spittle
五液	wǔ-yè	the five ye humors
脾阳	pí-yáng	the spleen-yang
虚弱	xū-ruò	depleted and weak
凝聚	níng-jù	congeal
成	chéng	become; form
痰饮	tán-yǐn	phlegm drink
上升	shàng-shēng	rise
干	gān	dry
欲	yù	wish
饮	yǐn	drink
温药	wēn-yào	warm(ing) drugs
缺少	quē-shǎo	deficiency
渴	kě	thirsty; thirst
口渴	kǒu-kě	thirst
热性病	rè-xìng-bìng	heat type illness

生津药	shēng-jīn-yào	drugs generating humor
石斛	shí-hú	(drug name) Dendrobium nobile Lindl.
麦冬	mài-dōng	(drug name) Ophiopogon japonicus Ker-Gawl.
玉竹	yù-zhú	(drug name) Polygonatum odoratum (Mill.) Druce and other Polygonatum species
天花粉	tiān-huā-fěn	(drug name) Trichosanthes kirilowii Maxim.
轻浅	qīng-qiǎn	mild; light
自	zì	self; automatic; spontaneous
回转	huí-zhuǎn	return
粘	nián	sticky
腻	nì	slimy
粘腻	nián-nì	sticky
考虑	kǎo-lǜ	consider
有无	yǒu-wú	whether or not
流弊	liú-bì	unwanted effects; drawback

Translation 5.8

The jin and ye humors can also transform into sweat, snivel, tears, saliva, and spittle. Basically, they are associated with the kidneys, and hence it is said that the kidneys rule the five ye humors. In persons whose spleen yang is depleted and weak, the humors do not transform. They may even congeal and collect and turn into phlegm-drink.[1] When phlegm-drink causes internal blocks, the humors have no (way) to rise. The mouth is dry, and (yet) there is no desire to drink. Warming drugs are to be employed to harmonize the (condition). A pathocondition of humor deficiency regularly witnessed in clinical practice is thirst. It is often caused by heat type illnesses. Drugs regularly employed to generate humors are, for instance, shihu, maidong, yuzhu, and tianhuafen. In cases of mild thirst, though, it is not necessary to use humor-generating drugs (in each and every case). The heat is cooled and the humors return by themselves. Humor generating drugs are often of a sticky and slimy nature; when applying them (therapists) should consider whether or not unwanted effects may accumulate over time. In severe cases of thirst that cannot be cured by generating humors, (therapists) must go a step further and apply, simultaneously, (drugs) that nourish the blood, and that nourish the yin.

Note

1 "Phlegm-drink" is a general designation for pathological fluids of different viscosities generated in the body during an illness. These fluids may be as thick as "phlegm" or as thin as a "drink."

Text 6.1

病因就是致病因素，分为内因，外因，不内外因三种。外因方面以六淫为主，即风，寒，暑，湿，燥，火。寒，暑，燥，湿，风本为一年四季的常气。在正常的情况下称为五气。又因暑即是热，热极能化火，其余风，湿，燥，寒在一定条件下亦能化火，因而又将"火"加入，一般称做"六气"。六气本为正常气候，亦称"正气"，如果非其时而有其气，便是反常气候，就叫"邪气"，如风邪，暑邪，湿邪之类，又因这种现象都是越出常轨，故又叫"六淫"。

Transliteration 6.1

Bìng-yīn jiù-shì zhì-bìng-yīn-sù, fēn-wéi nèi-yīn, wài-yīn, bú-nèi-wài-yīn sān zhǒng. Wài-yīn fāng-miàn yǐ liù-yín wéi zhǔ, jí fēng, hán, shǔ, shī, zào, huǒ. Hán, shǔ, zào, shī, fēng běn wéi yī nián sì-jì de cháng-qì. Zài zhèng-cháng de qíng-kuàng xià chēng-wéi wǔ-qì. Yòu yīn shǔ jí shì rè, rè jí néng huà huǒ, qí-yú fēng, shī, zào, hán zài yī-dìng tiáo-jiàn xià yì néng huà huǒ, yīn-ér yòu jiāng "huǒ" jiā-rù, yī-bān chēng-zuò "liù-qì." Liù-qì běn wéi zhèng-cháng qì-hòu, yì chēng "zhèng-qì," rú-guǒ fēi qí shí ér yǒu qí qì, biàn shì fǎn-cháng qì-hòu, jiù jiào "xié-qì," rú fēng-xié, shǔ-xié, shī-xié zhī lèi, yòu yīn zhè zhǒng xiàn-xiàng dōu-shì yuè-chū cháng guǐ, gù yòu jiào "liù-yín."

Vocabulary 6.1

病因	bìng-yīn	cause of illness
致病因素	zhì-bìng-yīn-sù	factors leading to illness
内因	nèi-yīn	internal causes
外因	wài-yīn	external causes
不内外因	bù-nèi-wài-yīn	neither internal nor external causes
... 方面	... fāng-miàn	as for ...
六淫	liù-yín	the six excesses
年	nián	year
四季	sì-jì	the four seasons
常气	cháng-qì	normal qi
五气	wǔ-qì	the five qi
极	jí	extreme

其余	qí-yú	the remaining
加入	jiā-rù	add
六气	liù-qì	the six qi
邪气	xié-qì	evil qi
风邪	fēng-xié	wind evil
暑邪	shǔ-xié	summerheat evil
湿邪	shī-xié	dampness evil
正气	zhèng-qì	proper qi
如果	rú-guǒ	if; when
越出	yuè-chū	transgress; leave
轨	guǐ	track; rails

Translation 6.1

Causes of illness are factors leading to illness; (Chinese medicine) distinguishes between the three types internal causes, external causes, and causes that are neither internal nor external. Among the external causes, it considers the six excesses as most important; they include wind, cold, summerheat, dampness, dryness, and fire. Basically, cold, summerheat, dryness, dampness, and wind are the regular qi of the four seasons in the course of one year. Under normal circumstances they are called the five qi. Since summerheat is heat, and since heat, when it is extreme, can turn into fire, and because under certain conditions wind, dampness, dryness, and cold can also turn into fire, (Chinese medicine) adds the "fire" (to the five qi) and speaks, in general, of "six qi." Basically, the six qi constitute the regular qi manifestations; they are also called "proper qi." If a specific qi appears when it is not its time, then this is an irregular qi manifestation. It is called "evil qi." Examples are wind evil, summerheat evil, or dampness evil. Furthermore, because such phenomena leave the normal course (of the seasons), they are also called the "six excesses."

Text 6.2

1. 风：风性多动善变，流行最广，常因季节不同，跟着气候转化，而有风温，风热，风寒之异。又常与其它邪气结合为风暑，风湿，风燥，风火等，故前人称风为百病之长。感染风邪发病，轻者在上焦气分为伤风，出现恶风，发热，头痛，鼻塞，流涕，咳嗽。重者在经络脏腑为"中风"，出现口眼歪斜，语言蹇涩，半身不遂，猝然倒仆，轻微的移时即能苏醒，严重的不省人事。

Transliteration 6.2

1. Fēng: fēng xìng duō dòng shàn biàn, liú-xíng zuì guǎng, cháng yīn jì-jié bù-tóng, gēn-zhe qì-hòu zhuǎn-huà, ér yǒu fēng-wēn, fēng-rè, fēng-hán zhī yì. Yòu cháng yǔ qí-tā xié-qì jié-hé wéi fēng-shǔ, fēng-shī, fēng-zào, fēng-huǒ děng, gù qián-rén chēng fēng wéi bǎi bìng zhī zhǎng. Gǎn-rǎn fēng-xié fā-bìng, qīng zhě zài shàng-jiāo qì-fèn wéi shāng-fēng, chū-xiàn wù-fēng, fā-rè, tóu-tòng, bí-sè, liú-tì, ké-sòu. Zhòng zhě zài jīng-luò zàng-fǔ wéi "zhòng-fēng," chū-xiàn kǒu yǎn wāi-xié, yǔ-yán jiǎn-sè, bàn-shēn-bù-suí, cù-rán dǎo-pū, qīng-wēi de yí-shí jí néng sū-xǐng, yán-zhòng de bù-xǐng-rén-shì.

Vocabulary 6.2

善	shàn	tend to
广	guǎng	wide
跟着	gēn-zhe	following
风温	fēng-wēn	wind-warmth
风热	fēng-rè	wind-heat
风暑	fēng-shǔ	wind-summerheat
风湿	fēng-shī	wind-dampness
风燥	fēng-zào	wind-dryness
风火	fēng-huǒ	wind-fire
长	zhǎng	chief
感染	gǎn-rǎn	affect; be affected by
恶风	wù-fēng	aversion to wind
流涕	liú-tì	flow of snivel
语言	yǔ-yán	speech
蹇涩	jiǎn-sè	impeded
半身不遂	bàn-shēn-bù-suí	hemiplegia
猝然	cù-rán	sudden
倒仆	dǎo-pū	collapse
轻微	qīng-wēi	mild; light
移	yí	move

移时	yí-shí	in the course of time
苏醒	sū-xǐng	regain consciousness
省	xǐng	recognize; know
不省人事	bù-xǐng-rén-shì	recognize neither people nor things

Translation 6.2

1. Wind: The nature of wind is frequent movement and a tendency to change; its passage covers the widest possible (regions). Because of the differences between the seasons, and following the changes of the climate, there are the different (combinations of) wind-warmth, wind-heat, and wind-cold. Also, (the wind) joins regularly with the other evil qi to form wind-summerheat, wind-dampness, wind-dryness, or wind-fire. Hence people in former times called the wind the chief (cause) of hundreds of illnesses. When affections by wind-evil provoke an illness, in minor cases this results in harm-caused-by-wind in the qi section of the upper burner, manifesting itself in aversion to wind, in fever, in headache, nasal obstruction, flow of snivel, and cough. In serious cases this is a "wind stroke" in the conduits and network (vessels, as well as) in the depots and bowels, manifesting itself in a wryness of mouth and eyes, in an impeded speech, in hemiplegia, and in sudden collapse. Mild (cases) will regain consciousness after some time; in serious (cases the patients) recognize neither people nor anything else.

Text 6.3

2. 寒：寒为阴邪，性主收引。伤于体表者为伤寒，呈现恶寒，发热，头痛，身体疼痛，脉象浮紧，舌苔白腻等症状。直接伤于里者为"中寒"，呈现呕吐清水，腹痛，肠鸣，大便泄泻，并有严重的肢冷，脉伏。祛散寒邪，只有辛温一法，但伤寒以解表为主，中寒则宜温中回阳。伤寒传变可以化热，不能固执温散，中寒很少化热，且常使阳气日渐衰退。

Transliteration 6.3

2. Hán: hán wéi yīn-xié, xìng zhǔ shōu-yǐn. Shāng yú tǐ-biǎo zhě wéi shāng-hán, chéng-xiàn wù-hán, fā-rè, tóu-tòng, shēn-tǐ téng-tòng, mài-xiàng fú jǐn, shé-tāi bái nì děng zhèng-zhuàng. Zhí-jiē shāng yú lǐ zhě wéi "zhòng-hán," chéng-xiàn ǒu-tù qīng-shuǐ, fù-tòng, cháng-míng, dà-biàn xiè-xiè, bìng yǒu yán-zhòng de zhī-lěng, mài fú. Qū sàn hán-xié, zhǐ-yǒu xīn-wēn yī fǎ, dàn shāng-hán yǐ jiě-biǎo wéi zhǔ, zhòng-hán zé yí wēn-zhōng huí-yáng. Shāng-hán chuán-biàn kě-yǐ huà rè, bù néng gù-zhí wēn sàn, zhòng-hán hěn shǎo huà rè, qiě cháng shǐ yáng-qì rì-jiàn shuāi-tuì.

Vocabulary 6.3

阴邪	yīn-xié	yin evil
收引	shōu-yǐn	draw together
伤寒	shāng-hán	harm caused by cold
呈现	chéng-xiàn	bring forth
恶寒	wù-hán	aversion to cold
脉象	mài-xiàng	pulse quality
紧	jǐn	tight
中寒	zhòng-hán	cold stroke
清水	qīng-shuǐ	clear water
腹痛	fù-tòng	abdominal pain
肠鸣	cháng-míng	intestinal sounds
肢冷	zhī-lěng	cold limbs
伏	fú	hide
祛	qū	dispell
辛温	xīn-wēn	acrid and warming
温中	wēn-zhōng	warm the center
回阳	huí-yáng	have the yang return
固执	gù-zhí	stubbornly cling to (something)
且	qiě	even
日渐	rì-jiàn	daily; day by day

Translation 6.3

2. Cold: Cold is a yin evil; its nature is chiefly to draw together. Harm at the body's outside is harm caused by cold; it brings forth pathoconditions such as aversion to cold, fever, headache, pain all over the body, a pulse that is near the surface and tight, and a white and oily coating of the tongue. Any harm directly affecting the interior is "cold stroke;" it brings forth (pathoconditions such as) clear liquid vomiting, abdominal pain, intestinal sounds, and diarrhea. In addition there are serious cases with limbs turning cold, and the pulse hiding away. For dispelling cold evil, there is only the one pattern of (using) acrid and warming (drugs). However, in case of harm caused by cold, it is most important to open the exterior, while in case of cold stroke it is appropriate to warm the center and have the yang return. When harm caused by cold is transmitted and transformed (in the body), it can change into heat, and (a therapy) must not stubbornly cling to warming and dispersing (patterns). A cold stroke very seldom changes into heat; on the contrary, it often causes the yang qi to weaken day by day.

3. 暑：暑是夏令的主气。暑病就是热病，仅是季节上的分别而已。故感受暑热，多见壮热，口渴，心烦，自汗等热症，由于暑热伤气，影响心脏，又常兼见喘喝，脉洪而虚。暑热挟风伤表，影响上焦，类似风温症初起，有恶风，身热，口渴，自汗等症。倘在烈日下长途奔走，或在田野劳动，感受暑热，则身热口渴，头痛，体重肢软，精神倦怠，小便短赤，这就称为中暑也叫中暍。暑热往往挟有湿气，这是由于天热地湿郁蒸的结果，或多啖瓜果，内先积湿，再感暑邪，则暑湿愈盛。

Transliteration 6.4

2. Shǔ: shǔ shì xià-lìng de zhǔ-qì. Shǔ-bìng jiù-shì rè-bìng, jǐn-shì jì-jié shàng-de fēn-bié ér-yǐ. Gù gǎn-shòu shǔ-rè, duō jiàn zhuàng-rè, kǒu-kě, xīn-fán, zì-hàn děng rè-zhèng, yóu-yú shǔ-rè shāng qì, yǐng-xiǎng xīn-zàng, yòu cháng jiān jiàn chuǎn-hè, mài hóng ér xū. Shǔ-rè xié fēng shāng biǎo, yǐng-xiǎng shàng-jiāo, lèi-sì fēng-wēn zhèng chū-qǐ, yǒu wù-fēng, shēn-rè, kǒu-kě, zì-hàn děng zhèng. Tǎng zài liè-rì xià cháng-tú bēn-zǒu, huò zài tián-yě láo-dòng, gǎn-shòu shǔ-rè, zé shēn-rè kǒu-kě, tóu-tòng, tǐ-zhòng zhī-ruǎn, jīng-shén juàn-dài, xiǎo-biàn-duǎn-chì, zhè jiù chēng-wéi zhòng-shǔ yě jiào zhòng-yè. Shǔ-rè wǎng-wǎng xié yǒu shī-qì, zhè shì yóu yú tiān rè dì shī yù-zhēng de jié-guǒ, huò duō dàn guā-guǒ, nèi xiān jī shī, zài gǎn shǔ-xié, zé shǔ-shī yù shèng.

Vocabulary 6.4

夏令	xià-lìng	summertime
主气	zhǔ-qì	ruling qi
暑病	shǔ-bìng	illnesses caused by summerheat
热病	rè-bìng	illnesses caused by heat
仅是 ... 而已	jǐn-shì ... ér-yǐ	be nothing but ...
感受	gǎn-shòu	be affected
暑热	shǔ-rè	summerheat-heat
壮热	zhuàng-rè	strong heat
心烦	xīn-fán	vexation of the heart
自汗	zì-hàn	spontaneous sweating
兼	jiān	together with

喘喝	chuǎn-hè	pant
洪	hóng	vast
挟	xié	in conjunction with
类似	lèi-sì	resemble
初起	chū-qǐ	begin
身热	shēn-rè	body heat
烈日	liè-rì	burning sun
长途	cháng-tú	long way; long distance
奔走	bēn-zǒu	walk
田野	tián-yě	open field
体重	tǐ-zhòng	heaviness of the body
肢软	zhī-ruǎn	soft limbs
倦怠	juàn-dài	fatigue
小便短赤	xiǎo-biàn-duǎn-chì	short voidings of reddish urine
中暑	zhòng-shǔ	summerheat stroke
中暍	zhòng-yè	sunstroke
湿气	shī-qì	dampness qi
地	dì	soil
郁蒸	yù-zhēng	heavy steaming
结果	jié-guǒ	result
啖	dàn	eat
瓜果	guā-guǒ	gourds
积	jī	accumulate
感	gǎn	be affected
暑湿	shǔ-shī	summerheat-dampness
愈	yù	even more

Translation 6.4

3. Summerheat: Summerheat is the ruling qi of summertime. Summerheat illnesses are heat illnesses; the distinction (between heat and summerheat) is based only on the seasons (during which they occur). Hence in case of an affection by summerheat-heat, often witnessed heat pathoconditions are strong heat, thirst, vexation of the heart, and spontaneous sweating. Since

harm caused to the qi by the heat of summerheat has an effect on the heart, panting and a vast and depleted pulse are observed regularly in addition. When summerheat-heat harms the (the body's) exterior in conjunction with wind, this affects the upper burner, and in the beginning pathoconditions resembling wind warmth appear. These are pathoconditions such as aversion to wind, body heat, thirst, and spontaneous sweating. When (a person) walks a long way under the burning sun, or toils out in the fields, and is affected by the heat of summerheat, this will result in body heat, thirst, headache, heaviness of the body, soft limbs, mental fatigue, and short voidings of reddish urine. Such (a condition) is called summerheat stroke; is is also called sunstroke. Summerheat heat occurs often in conjunction with dampness qi. In such a case as a result of heavy steaming caused by a hot sky and a damp earth, or because of a repeated consumption of gourds dampness has accumulated in the interior first to which was added an affection by summerheat evil, so that summerheat dampness (is present in the body) in even greater abundance.

4. 湿：湿为重浊之邪，粘滞难化。在外因中多指雾露或天雨潮湿，感受者发为寒热，鼻塞，骨节酸疼。也有因坐卧湿地，居处潮湿，或水中作业，汗出沾衣，湿邪由皮肤流入肌肉，经络，则发生浮肿和关节疼痛等症。嗜食膏粱厚味，或过食生冷瓜果，甜腻食品，能使脾阳不运，湿自内生，称做内湿。内湿在上则为胸闷，气分不畅，痰多；在中则为脘痞，呕吐，消化不良；在下则为腹满，溲少，大便泄泻；也能上至头为面浮，下至足为脚肿。

Transliteration 6.5

4. Shī: shī wéi zhòng zhuó zhī xié, nián zhì nán huà. Zài wài-yīn zhōng duō zhǐ wù lù huò tiān-yǔ cháo-shī, gǎn-shòu zhě fā wéi hán rè, bí-sè, gǔ jié suān-téng. Yě yǒu yīn zuò wò shī dì, jū chù cháo-shī, huò shuǐ zhōng zuò-yè, hàn-chū zhān yī, shī-xié yóu pí-fū liú-rù jī-ròu, jīng-luò, zé fā-shēng fú-zhǒng hé guān-jié téng-tòng děng zhèng. Shì shí gāo-liáng hòu wèi, huò guò shí shēng lěng guā-guǒ, tián nì shí-pǐn, néng shǐ pí-yáng bù yùn, shī zì nèi shēng, chēng-zuò nèi-shī. Nèi-shī zài shàng zé wéi xiōng-mèn, qì-fèn bù chàng, tán duō; zài zhōng zé wéi wǎn-pǐ, ǒu-tù, xiāo-huà bù liáng, zài xià zé wéi fù-mǎn, sōu-shǎo, dà-biàn xiè-xiè; yě néng shàng zhì tóu wéi miàn fú, xià zhì zú wéi jiǎo-zhǒng.

Vocabulary 6.5

难	nán	difficult
雾	wù	fog
露	lù	dew
天雨	tiān-yǔ	rain
潮湿	cháo-shī	moisture
发	fā	develop; bring forth
节	jié	joint
坐	zuò	sit
卧	wò	lie down
居	jū	live
作业	zuò-yè	work
沾	zhān	wet

衣	yī	clothing
皮肤	pí-fū	skin
流入	liú-rù	flow into
嗜	shì	take delight in
膏粱	gāo-liáng	rich food
厚	hòu	thick; rich in contents
过	guò	excessive; too much
甜	tián	sweet
食品	shí-pǐn	food items
内湿	nèi-shī	internal dampness
痰	tán	phlegm
脘	wǎn	(stomach) duct
脘痞	wǎn-pǐ	blockage of the (stomach) duct
不良	bù-liáng	not good; bad
腹满	fù-mǎn	abdominal fullness
溲少	sōu-shǎo	scant urine
面	miàn	face
浮	fú	bloated
脚肿	jiǎo-zhǒng	swollen legs

Translation 6.5

4. Dampness: Dampness is the evil of heaviness and turbidity; it is sticky and sluggish, and does not transform itself easily. Among the external causes (of illness, dampness) often refers to the moisture of fog and dew, or of rain. Those affected (by this evil) develop (alternating) cold and heat, nasal obstruction, and pain in bones and joints. It also happens because (a person) sits or lies at a damp place, or lives in a moist (environment), or works in water, or because sweat leaves (the body) and wettens the clothes that dampness evil flows from the skin into the flesh, and into the conduits and network (vessels), and then develops pathoconditions such as edematous swelling, and pain in the joints. If someone takes delight in eating rich food, or consumes too much raw and cold (foods like) gourds and fruits, as well as sweet and greasy foods, that

may cause the yang (qi) of the spleen not to move, and dampness to emerge internally. This is called internal dampness. When internal dampness is situated in the upper (region of the body), then this causes chest pressure. The qi section is not free; (it is blocked by) lots of phlegm. When it is situated in the center, then this brings about blockage of the (stomach) duct, vomiting, and poor digestion. When it is situated in the lower (region), then this causes (a feeling of) fullness in the abdomen, oliguria, and diarrhea. It can also rise to the head and cause facial bloating, or it may descend into the feet and cause swollen legs.

5. 燥：燥为秋季主气，亦称秋燥。外感秋燥之邪多在上焦，类似伤风，表现为微寒微热，头痛，口干，唇干，鼻干，咽喉干，干咳无痰，或痰少粘滞挟血，大便燥结等。燥亦为火之余气，热病之后往往发现干燥现象。燥与津血又有密切关系，津血内亏，燥症易起。凡此皆属内伤，不同秋燥时气外乘，故秋燥当于甘凉剂中佐入微辛清泄，此则但宜甘凉清润。内伤燥症范围较广，在外则皮肤干糙，口唇燥裂，目涩；在内则渴饮，善饥，咽干噎膈，便闭，尿黄短涩等。

Transliteration 6.6

5. Zào: zào wéi qiū-jì zhǔ-qì, yì chēng qiū-zào. Wài-gǎn qiū-zào zhī xié duō zài shàng-jiāo, lèi-sì shāng-fēng, biǎo-xiàn wéi wēi hán wēi rè, tóu-tòng, kǒu gān, chún gān, bí gān, yān-hóu gān, gān-ké wú tán, huò tán shǎo nián zhì xié xuè, dà-biàn zào jié děng. Zào yì wéi huǒ zhī yú-qì, rè-bìng zhī-hòu wǎng-wǎng fā-xiàn gān-zào xiàn-xiàng. Zào yǔ jīn xuè yòu yǒu mì-qiè guān-xi, jīn xuè nèi kuī, zào-zhèng yì qǐ. Fán cǐ jiē shǔ nèi-shāng, bù-tóng qiū-zào shí-qì wài-chéng, gù qiū-zào dāng yú gān-liáng-jì zhōng zuǒ rù wēi xīn qīng xiè, cǐ zé dàn yí gān liáng qīng rùn. Nèi-shāng zào-zhèng fàn-wéi jiào guǎng, zài wài zé pí-fū gān cāo, kǒu chún zào-liè, mù sè; zài nèi zé kě-yǐn, shàn jī, yān-gān yē-gé, biàn-bì, niào huáng duǎn sè děng.

Vocabulary 6.6

秋季	qiū-jì	autumn
秋燥	qiū-zào	autumn dryness
外感	wài-gǎn	external affection
表现	biǎo-xiàn wéi	become manifest as
微	wēi	little
唇	chún	lip
干咳	gān-ké	dry coughing
咽喉	yān-hóu	throat
结	jié	knot; cloddy
余气	yú-qì	residual qi
之后	zhī-hòu	following; after
干燥	gān-zào	dryness

亏	kuī	loss
燥症	zào-zhèng	dryness pathoconditions
内伤	nèi-shāng	internal harm
时气	shí-qì	seasonal qi
外乘	wài-chéng	external affection
甘凉剂	gān-liáng-jì	sweet and cooling formula
润	rùn	moist; moisten
范围	fàn-wéi	spectrum
较	jiào	relatively; comparatively
糙	cāo	coarse
燥裂	zào-liè	dry out and crack
渴饮	kě-yǐn	thirst
饥	jī	be hungry; hunger
咽干	yān-gān	dry throat
噎膈	yē-gé	esophageal constriction
便闭	biàn-bì	constipation
短	duǎn	short; (in the present context in conjunction with the character niao [urine]:) scant urine

Translation 6.6

5. Dryness: Dryness is the ruling qi of autumn; it is also called autumn dryness. An external affection by the evil of autumn dryness often occurs in the upper burner, and resembles (in its effects) harm caused by wind. It manifests itself as mild cold (alternating with) mild heat, headache, dry mouth, dry lips, dry nose, dry throat, dry coughing without phlegm, or with a little phlegm that is sticky and sluggish and that is mixed with blood, as well as dry and cloddy stool. Dryness is also a residual qi of fire; dryness phenomena often develop following heat illnesses. Dryness is also closely related to the jin humors and the blood. When the jin humors or the blood are lost internally, dryness pathoconditions emerge easily. All these (conditions) belong to internal harm, and are unlike external affections with the seasonal qi of autumn dryness. Hence in case of autumn dryness

sweet and cooling formulas must be amended by slightly acrid (substances) to achieve cooling and draining. (For the inner harm mentioned) here, though, it is appropriate only to use sweet and cooling (substances) to cool and moisten. The spectrum of dryness pathoconditions (resulting from) inner harm is relatively broad; externally (they include the following:) the skin is dry and coarse, the mouth and the lips dry out and crack, and the eyes become rough. Internally (they include) thirst and hunger, a dry throat, esophageal blockage, constipation, as well as scant yellow urine that is rough (in its flow).

6. 火：从外因方面来说，火是一种热邪，由风，寒，暑，燥，湿五气所化。及其燔灼则充斥三焦，表现为口臭，喉痛红肿，胸闷烦躁，腹满溲赤，甚至发斑发疹，神昏狂乱，迫血妄行，有如燎原之势。五脏亦能化火，称做五志之火。以肝胆之火最为多见，症现目赤，口苦，头昏胀痛，面红耳鸣，睡眠不安，乱梦颠倒，胸闷，以及梦遗，淋浊等。不论五气化火或五志之火，多为实火，当用苦寒直折，不是一般清热剂所能治疗。

Transliteration 6.7

6. Huǒ: cóng wài-yīn fāng-miàn lái shuō, huǒ shì yī zhǒng rè-xié, yóu fēng, hán, shǔ, zào, shī wǔ-qì suǒ huà. Jí qí fán-zhuó zé chōng-chì sān-jiāo, biǎo-xiàn wéi kǒu-chòu, hóu tòng hóng zhǒng, xiōng-mèn fán-zào, fù-mǎn sōu chì, shèn-zhì fā-bān fā-zhěn, shén-hūn kuáng-luàn, pò xuè wàng xíng, yǒu rú liáo-yuán zhī shì. Wǔ-zàng yì néng huà huǒ, chēng-zuò wǔ-zhì zhī huǒ. Yǐ gān dǎn zhī huǒ zuì-wéi duō jiàn, zhèng xiàn mù-chì, kǒu-kǔ, tóu-hūn zhàng-tòng, miàn hóng ěr-míng, shuì-mián bù-ān, luàn mèng diān-dǎo, xiōng-mèn, yǐ-jí mèng-yí, lín-zhuó děng. Bù-lùn wǔ-qì huà huǒ huò wǔ-zhì zhī huǒ, duō wéi shí-huǒ, dāng yòng kǔ hán zhí zhé, bù shì yī-bān qīng-rè jì suǒ néng zhì-liáo.

Vocabulary 6.7

燔灼	fán-zhuó	burn
充斥	chōng-chì	fill
口臭	kǒu-chòu	bad breath
喉	hóu	throat
烦躁	fán-zào	vexation
溲	sōu	urinate; urine
发斑	fā-bān	develop macules
发疹	fā-zhěn	develop pustules
神昏	shén-hūn	mental confusion
狂乱	kuáng-luàn	wild behavior
迫	pò	agitated
行	xíng	move
燎原	liáo-yuán	prairie fire
势	shì	force
最为	zuì-wéi	be most... (to express superlative)
目赤	mù-chì	red eyes
头昏	tóu-hūn	clouded head
胀痛	zhàng-tòng	pressure and pain

睡眠	shuì-mián	sleep
不安	bù-ān	restless; unquiet
乱	luàn	wild
梦	mèng	dream
颠倒	diān-dǎo	confusion
梦遗	mèng-yí	dream emission
淋浊	lín-zhuó	strangury and turbid (urine)
实火	shí-huǒ	repletion fire
直	zhí	direct
折	zhé	break
剂	jì	formula

Translation 6.7

6. Fire: Mentioned in the context of external causes (of illness), fire is a type of heat evil resulting from a transformation of any of the five qi, (namely) wind, cold, summerheat, dryness, and dampness. When it burns, it fills the triple burner. Manifestations are bad breath, painful, red, and swollen throat, a feeling of pressure in the chest, and vexation, abdominal fullness, and reddish urine. Serious cases develop pustules and macules, mental confusion and wild behavior, as well as disorderly movement of agitated blood, with (all these conditions) having the force of a prairie fire. The five depots can also produce fire through transformation. This is called the fire of the five minds. The fire of liver and gall can be observed most often. Red eyes, a bitter (taste in the) mouth, clouded head, pressure, and pain in the head, a red face and sounds in the ears, broken sleep, wild dreams and confusion, pressure in the chest as well as dream emissions, and strangury as well as turbid (urine) appear as pathoconditions. No matter whether it is a fire resulting from a transformation of any of the five qi, or whether it is a fire of the five minds, it is mostly a repletion fire, and bitter and cold (drugs) must be employed to cut it directly. It cannot be healed by common formulas cooling heat.

Text 6.8

感染六淫之邪不即发病，经过一个相当时期方才出现病症，例如，冬天受了寒邪，到夏天才生温病；夏天受了暑邪，到秋天才出现暑病。这就称做"伏邪"。疫疠之邪，亦为外来致病因素之一。疫是互相染易，不问大小，病状相似，即传染的意思；疠是指自然界一种毒戾之气，危害健康最大，不同于普通的六淫之邪。疠气的发生，多由淫雨，亢旱，或家畜瘟死，秽物腐败等酝酿所成。从性质上分为寒疫和瘟疫两项，多由口鼻吸受，直入肠胃，发病极速。

Transliteration 6.8

Gǎn-rǎn liù-yín zhī xié bù jí fā-bìng, jīng-guò yī-gè xiāng-dāng shí-qī fāng-cái chū-xiàn bìng-zhèng, lì-rú, dōng-tiān shòu le hán-xié, dào xià-tiān cái shēng wēn-bìng; xià-tiān shòu le shǔ-xié, dào qiū-tiān cái chū-xiàn shǔ-bìng. Zhè jiù chēng-zuò "fú-xié." Yì-lì zhī xié, yì wéi wài lái zhì-bìng-yīn-sù zhī-yī. Yì shì hù-xiāng rǎn yì, bù-wèn dà-xiǎo, bìng-zhuàng xiāng-sì, jí chuán-rǎn de yì-si; lì shì zhǐ zì-rán-jiè yī zhǒng dú-lì zhī qì, wēi-hài jiàn-kāng zuì dà, bù-tóng yú pǔ-tōng de liù-yín zhī xié. Lì qì de fā-shēng, duō yóu yín-yǔ, kàng-hàn, huò jiā-chù wēn sǐ, huì wù fǔ-bài děng yùn-niàng suǒ chéng. Cóng xìng-zhì shàng fēn-wéi hán-yì hé wēn-yì liǎng xiàng, duō yóu kǒu bí xī-shòu, zhí rù cháng wèi, fā-bìng jí-sù.

Vocabulary 6.8

即	jí	immediately
经过	jīng-guò	pass
相当	xiāng-dāng	relative; certain
时期	shí-qī	period of time
方才	fāng-cái	then
冬天	dōng-tiān	winter
夏天	xià-tiān	summer
温病	wēn-bìng	warmth illness
秋天	qiū-tiān	autumn
伏邪	fú-xié	hidden evil
疫疠	yì-lì	epidemics
染	rǎn	infect

不问	bù-wèn	regardless whether
大小	dà-xiǎo	size; age
病状	bìng-zhuàng	appearance of an illness
传染	chuán-rǎn	infection through transmission
毒戾	dú-lì	pernicious
危害	wēi-hài	dangerous
健康	jiàn-kāng	health
普通	pǔ-tōng	general
淫雨	yín-yǔ	excessive rain
亢旱	kàng-hàn	severe drought
家	jiā	house; family
家畜	jiā-chù	livestock
瘟	wēn	infectious disease
死	sǐ	die
秽	huì	filth; dirty matter
腐败	fǔ-bài	decay; rot
酝酿	yùn-niàng	ferment
寒疫	hán-yì	cold epidemics
温疫	wēn-yì	warmth epidemics
吸	xī	inhale
吸受	xī-shòu	take in through inhalation
极速	jí-sù	very fast

Translation 6.8

An affection by an evil of the six excesses does not bring forth an illness immediately. Illness conditions will appear only after a certain period of time has passed. For example, if someone has received a cold evil in winter, this will generate a warmth illness in summer. If someone has received a summerheat evil in summer, this will develop a summerheat illness in autumn. This is called "hidden evil." The evils of epidemics constitute further external factors causing illness. (Of the two characters yì-lì constituting the term epidemics, the first character, i.e.,) yì means "to pass (an illness) from one to another," with the appearances of the illness resembling each other (in each consecutive patient) regardless whether it is an adult or a child. (The second character, i.e.,) lì refers to a pernicious qi of the natural world, with great danger for (the patient's) health; it is not like the common evil of the six excesses. The emergence of pernicious qi is mostly a result of excessive rain or severe drought, or of fermentations (resulting from) the death of livestock because of an infectious disease, or from the rotting of dirty matter. With respect to their nature, the two types of cold epidemics and warmth epidemics are distinguished. They are mostly inhaled through mouth and nose, and enter directly into the intestines and the stomach where they develop an illness very quickly.

Text 7.1

内因以七情为主，还有痰，瘀，寄生虫等，同为重要因素。

1. 七情：七情即忧，思，喜，怒，悲，恐，惊。七情发病是一种情志病，是因于外界事物的刺激，使精神上发生变化。由于外界刺激的不同，精神的变化也有不同的反映。常见的症状，如抑郁不乐，喜怒无常，心烦意乱，惊惕善疑，失眠多梦，悲哀哭泣，不饥不食，胸闷太息，严重的神志恍惚，语言错乱，如癫如痴。七情引起的病变，主要是气的变化。总的说来，七情的影响最先是气，气与血是不可分离的，故病情进一步就影响到血。

Transliteration 7.1

Nèi-yīn yǐ qī-qíng wéi zhǔ, hái-yǒu tán, yū, jì-shēng-chóng děng, tóng wéi zhòng-yào yīn-sù.

1. Qī-qíng: Qī-qíng jí yōu, sī, xǐ, nù, bēi, kǒng, jīng. Qī-qíng fā-bìng shì yī zhǒng qíng-zhì-bìng, shì yīn yú wài-jiè shì-wù de cì-jī, shǐ jīng-shén shàng fā-shēng biàn-huà. Yóu-yú wài-jiè cì-jī de bù-tóng, jīng-shén de biàn-huà yě yǒu bù-tóng de fǎn-yìng. Cháng jiàn de zhèng-zhuàng, rú yì-yù bù-lè, xǐ nù wú-cháng, xīn-fán yì-luàn, jīng-tì shàn yí, shī-mián duō mèng, bēi-āi kū-qì, bù jī bù shí, xiōng-mèn tài-xī, yán-zhòng de shén-zhì huǎng-hū, yǔ-yán cuò-luàn, rú diān rú chī. Qī-qíng yǐn-qǐ de bìng-biàn, zhǔ-yào shì qì de biàn-huà. Zǒng-de-shuō-lái, qī-qíng de yǐng-xiǎng zuì xiān shì qì, qì yǔ xuè shì bù-kě fēn-lí de, gù bìng-qíng jìn-yī-bù jiù yǐng-xiǎng dào xuè.

Vocabulary 7.1

七情	qī-qíng	seven affects
寄生虫	jì-shēng-chóng	parasite
悲	bēi	sorrow
惊	jīng	fright
情志病	qíng-zhì-bìng	emotional illness

抑郁	yì-yù	depression
不乐	bù-lè	discontent
无常	wú-cháng	irregular
意乱	yì-luàn	mental chaos
疑	yí	doubt
悲哀	bēi-āi	grief
哭泣	kū-qì	cry
太息	tài-xī	deep sigh
神志	shén-zhì	mind
恍惚	huǎng-hū	absentminded
错乱	cuò-luàn	uncontrolled
癫	diān	insanity
痴	chī	idiocy
总的说来	zǒng-de-shuō-lái	generally speaking
病情	bìng-qíng	illness

Translation 7.1

The seven affects are the major internal causes (of illness); in addition, phlegm, stagnations, and parasites are important factors.

1. The seven affects: The seven affects are anxiety, thought, joy, anger, sorrow, fear, and fright. The illnesses brought forth by the seven affects are a kind of emotional illness; they are changes that have developed in the mind as a result of a stimulus by some environmental entity. Because the environmental stimuli (affecting man may) differ, the (corresponding) changes of the mind differ too. Often seen illness manifestations (include), for instance, depression with discontent, irregular joy and anger, vexation and mental chaos, suspicion and a tendency to doubt, insomnia with frequent dreams, grief with tearflow, loss of appetite and no consumption of food, and a feeling of pressure in the chest accompanied by deep sighs. Serious cases include absentmindedness and uncontrolled speech, resembling insanity or idiocy. The pathological changes evoked by the seven affects are mainly transformations of qi. Generally speaking, the seven affects influence the qi first. Since the qi and the blood are linked inseparably, the illness will then influence the blood.

Text 7.2

七情变化既由外界刺激引起，似可作为外因，但是与一般的外因发病毕竟不一样。外因引起的只要去其外因其病即愈，七情已经在精神上起到变化，并使内在的生活情况改变，即使刺激不再存在时也不能立即恢复。同样的七情病，由于刺激有强弱，在病症上就有显著的差别。同时，病人的体质和敏感性，对受病亦有极大关系，需要仔细观察。

Transliteration 7.2

Qī-qíng biàn-huà jí yóu wài-jiè cì-jī yǐn-qǐ, sì kě zuò-wéi wài-yīn, dàn-shì yǔ yī-bān de wài-yīn fā-bìng bì-jìng bù yī-yàng. Wài-yīn yǐn-qǐ de zhǐ yào qù qí wài-yīn qí bìng jí yù, qī-qíng yǐ-jīng zài jīng-shén shàng qǐ dào biàn-huà, bìng shǐ nèi-zài de shēng-huó qíng-kuàng gǎi-biàn, jí shǐ cì-jī bù-zài cún-zài shí yě bù néng lì-jí huī-fù. Tóng-yàng de qī-qíng-bìng, yóu-yú cì-jī yǒu qiáng-ruò, zài bìng-zhèng shàng jiù yǒu xiǎn-zhù de chā-bié. Tóng-shí, bìng-rén de tǐ-zhì hé mǐn-gǎn-xìng, duì shòu bìng yì yǒu jí-dà guān-xi, xū-yào zǐ-xì guān-chá.

Vocabulary 7.2

毕竟	bì-jìng	finally; in the final analysis
只	zhǐ	only
内在	nèi-zài	internal
生活	shēng-huó	life
改变	gǎi-biàn	change
即使 ... 也不 ...	jí shǐ ... yě bù ...	even if ... nevertheless not ...
不再	bù-zài	not again; not any longer
立即	lì-jí	immediate
七情病	qī-qíng-bìng	illnesses (caused) by the seven affects
显著	xiǎn-zhù	obvious
差别	chā-bié	difference
病人	bìng-rén	sick person; patient
敏感性	mǐn-gǎn-xìng	susceptibility; sensitivity
极大	jí-dà	very big
仔细	zǐ-xì	carefully

Translation 7.2

Since the changes in the seven affects are caused by environmental stimuli, it seems as if the (latter) could be regarded as external causes (of illness). In the final analysis, though, (the way these environmental stimuli give rise to illness) differs from how the common external causes give rise to an illness. In case of (illnesses) brought forth by external causes, all there is to do is to remove the external cause, and the illness will be cured. When the seven affects have already brought about changes in the mind, though, and when, furthermore, they have stimulated changes in the internal physiological conditions, an elimination of the stimulus cannot result in an immediate recovery (of the patient). Identical illnesses (caused by any) of the seven affects will show obvious differences in their manifestations because the (environmental) stimulus may have been strong or weak. At the same time, the patient's constitution and susceptibility are also closely related to a contraction of an illness, and have to be carefully examined.

2. 痰：脾阳衰弱，水湿不化，凝聚成痰；肺热煎熬津液，亦能成痰。痰与内脏的关系，以肺和脾最为密切。痰的主要症状为咳嗽，阻碍气机肃降则为喘息；亦能流窜经络，出现手足麻木，舌强蹇涩，瘰疬瘿瘤等症。若和其它因素结合，有寒痰，热痰，燥痰，湿痰，风痰等，则症状更为复杂了。痰在病因中占有重要地位，除了因痰生病之外，很多病症均能引起痰浊，既有痰浊必须兼顾。

Transliteration 7.3

2. Tán: pí-yáng shuāi-ruò, shuǐ-shī bù huà, níng-jù chéng tán; fèi-rè jiān-áo jīn-yè, yì néng chéng tán. Tán yǔ nèi-zàng de guān-xi, yǐ fèi hé pí zuì wéi mì-qiè. Tán de zhǔ-yào zhèng-zhuàng wéi ké-sòu, zǔ-ài qì-jī sù jiàng zé wéi chuǎn-xī; yì néng liú-cuàn jīng-luò, chū-xiàn shǒu zú má-mù, shé-jiàng jiǎn-sè, luǒ-lì yǐng-liú děng zhèng. Ruò hé qí-tā yīn-sù jié-hé, yǒu hán-tán, rè-tán, zào-tán, shī-tán, fēng-tán děng, zé zhèng-zhuàng gèng wéi fù-zá le. Tán zài bìng-yīn zhōng zhàn-yǒu zhòng-yào dì-wèi, chú-le yīn tán shēng bìng zhī wài, hěn duō bìng-zhèng jūn néng yǐn-qǐ tán-zhuó, jí yǒu tán-zhuó bì-xū jiān-gù.

Vocabulary 7.3

肺热	fèi-rè	lung heat
煎熬	jiān-áo	boil
阻碍	zǔ-ài	block
肃	sù	free; unimpeded
喘息	chuǎn-xī	pant
流窜	liú-cuàn	flow through ...
瘰疬	luǒ-lì	scrofula
瘿瘤	yǐng-liú	goiter
若	ruò	if; when
寒痰	hán-tán	cold-phlegm
热痰	rè-tán	heat-phlegm
燥痰	zào-tán	dryness-phlegm
湿痰	shī-tán	dampness-phlegm
风痰	fēng-tán	wind-phlegm
复杂	fù-zá	complex; complicated
占有	zhàn-yǒu	have
地位	dì-wèi	position
除了	chú-le	except for
痰浊	tán-zhuó	phlegm-turbidity
顾	gù	observe

兼顾	jiān-gù	take into regard simultaneously

Translation 7.3

2. Phlegm: When the yang (qi) of the spleen is weak, the liquids (that are consumed) are not transformed. They coagulate and generate phlegm. When the heat of the lung causes the body fluids to boil, this too may generate phlegm. Of the relationships between phlegm and the internal depots, those with the lung and with the spleen are the closest. The major pathological manifestation brought forth by phlegm is cough. When (phlegm) blocks the unimpeded downward dynamics of the qi, then this causes panting. (Phlegm) can also flow through the conduits and network (vessels), and cause pathoconditions such as numbness of hands and feet, heaviness and laming of the tongue, as well as scrofula and goiter. When (phlegm) and the other (illness causing) factors merge, there may be cold phlegm, heat phlegm, dryness phlegm, dampness phlegm, and wind phlegm, and the pathoconditions become even more complex. Phlegm occupies an important position among the causes of illness. In addition to illnesses generated by phlegm, very many illnesses can give rise to phlegm-turbidity. Hence when phlegm turbidity is present, this (possibility) must be taken into account too.

Text 7.4

3. 饮食：饮食为营养的泉源，但恣贪口腹，没有节制，运化不及，亦能致病。如胸膈痞闷，脘腹胀痛，吐逆吞酸，或引起寒热，头痛，泄泻的，称做伤食。伤食，多成肠胃病。也有本身消化薄弱，不能多食，食后饱胀，稍进油腻，大便溏薄，中医称为脾虚。并以能食不消化为胃强脾弱，知饥不能食为脾强胃弱。

Transliteration 7.4

3. Yǐn-shí: yǐn-shí wéi yíng yǎng de quán-yuán, dàn zì tān kǒu-fù, méi-yǒu jié-zhì, yùn-huà bù-jí, yì néng zhì-bìng. Rú xiōng gé pǐ-mèn, wǎn fù zhàng tòng, tǔ-nì tūn-suān, huò yǐn-qǐ hán rè, tóu-tòng, xiè-xiè de, chēng-zuò shāng-shí. Shāng-shí, duō chéng cháng-wèi-bìng. Yě yǒu běn-shēn xiāo-huà bó-ruò, bù néng duō shí, shí hòu bǎo zhàng, shāo jìn yóu nì, dà-biàn táng-

bó, zhōng-yī chēng-wéi pí-xū. Bìng yǐ néng shí bù xiāo-huà wéi wèi qiáng pí ruò, zhī-jī bù néng shí wéi pí qiáng wèi ruò.

Vocabulary 7.4

泉源	quán-yuán	source
恣	zì	unrestrained
贪	tān	gluttonous
口腹	kǒu-fù	eat; consume
节制	jié-zhì	restrain
运化	yùn-huà	movement and transformation; digestion
致病	zhì-bìng	lead to illness
痞闷	pǐ-mèn	blocks and chest pressure
腹	fù	abdomen
吐逆	tǔ-nì	vomit
吞酸	tūn-suān	acid regurgitation
伤食	shāng-shí	harm (caused by) food
肠胃病	cháng-wèi-bìng	illnesses of the intestines and of the stomach
本身	běn-shēn	by nature
薄弱	bó-ruò	weak
饱	bǎo	full (after eating); bloated
进	jìn	move into; eat
油	yóu	oil; oily
溏薄	táng-bó	semiliquid
脾虚	pí-xū	spleen depletion
饥	jī	be hungry; hunger

Translation 7.4

3. Food and Drink: Food and drink are the sources of nourishment. However, indulgence in food without restraint, as well as inadequate

digestion, can also lead to illness. For example, blocks and a feeling of pressure in the chest and at the diaphragm, swelling and pain in the stomach duct or in the abdomen, vomiting and acid regurgitation, or such (problems) that may give rise to fits of alternating cold and heat, to headache, or diarrhea, they are called harm (caused by) food. Harm (caused by) food mostly generates illnesses of the intestines and of the stomach. It may also be that the digestion (of the patient's stomach) was weak by nature. (The patient) cannot eat much, and after meals feels full and distended. If only small amounts of oily or greasy food are consumed, the stools will be semiliquid. Chinese medicine calls this spleen depletion. Also, it considers an ability to eat coupled with an absence of digestion as (an indication of) a strong stomach accompanied by a weak spleen, while it recognizes hunger coupled with an inability to eat as a strong spleen accompanied by a weak stomach.

4. 虫：以蛔虫，蛲虫，寸白虫等肠寄生虫为常见。多由湿热素重，饮食不洁，杂进生菜瓜果和香燥肥甘等而成。患有肠寄生虫病的症状，呈现面黄肌瘦，眼眶，鼻下黑色，鼻孔或肛门作痒，唇内生白点如粟粒，食欲减退或异常亢进，有的还嗜食生米，茶叶，腹内阵痛，面部变色。在小儿尤易酿成疳积，腹大坚满，俗呼疳膨食积。痨瘵即传尸痨，由痨虫传染，病在于肺。症见咳嗽咯血，失音气促，骨蒸盗汗，面色皓白，颧红如妆，伤人最甚。

Transliteration 7.5

4. Chóng: yǐ huí-chóng, náo-chóng, cùn-bái-chóng děng cháng jì-shēng-chóng wéi cháng jiàn. Duō yóu shī-rè sù zhòng, yǐn-shí bù jié, zá jìn shēng cài guā-guǒ hé xiāng zào féi gān děng ér chéng. Huàn yǒu cháng jì-shēng-chóng bìng de zhèng-zhuàng, chéng-xiàn miàn huáng jī shòu, yǎn-kuàng, bí xià hēi sè, bí-kǒng huò gāng-mén zuò-yǎng, chún nèi shēng bái diǎn rú sù-lì, shí-yù jiǎn-tuì huò yì-cháng kàng-jìn, yǒu-de hái shì shí shēng mǐ, chá-yè, fù nèi zhèn-tòng, miàn-bù biàn sè. Zài xiǎo-ér yóu yì niàng-chéng gān-jī, fù dà jiān mǎn, sú hū gān péng shí-jī. Láo-zhài jí chuán-shī-láo, yóu láo-chóng chuán-rǎn, bìng zài yú fèi. Zhèng jiàn ké-sòu kǎ-xuè, shī-yīn qì-cù, gǔ-zhēng dào-hàn, miàn-sè hào-bái, quán hóng rú zhuāng, shāng rén zuì shèn.

Vocabulary 7.5

虫	chóng	worm
蛔虫	huí-chóng	roundworm
蛲虫	náo-chóng	pinworm
寸白虫	cùn-bái-chóng	tapeworm
湿热	shī-rè	dampness and heat
素	sù	permanent
洁	jié	clean
杂	zá	various; mixed
菜	cài	vegetables
香	xiāng	aromatic; fragrant
肥	féi	fat

瘦	shòu	emaciated
眼眶	yǎn-kuàng	eye socket
鼻孔	bí-kǒng	nostril
肛门	gāng-mén	anus
作痒	zuò-yǎng	itch
点	diǎn	spot
粟粒	sù-lì	millet grain
食欲	shí-yù	appetite
减退	jiǎn-tuì	decrease
异常	yì-cháng	abnormal
有的	yǒu-de	some
米	mǐ	rice
茶叶	chá-yè	tea leaves
阵痛	zhèn-tòng	the pains of birth
面部	miàn-bù	face
小儿	xiǎo-ér	small children
尤	yóu	especially
酿成	niàng-chéng	develop
疳积	gān-jī	malnutrition accumulation
坚	jiān	hard; solid
满	mǎn	fullness; full
俗	sú	commonly
呼	hū	call
膨	péng	inflation
食积	shí-jī	food accumulation
痨瘵	láo-zhài	consumption
传尸痨	chuán-shī-láo	consumption transmitted by corpses
痨虫	láo-chóng	consumption worms
咯血	kǎ-xuè	haemoptysis
失音	shī-yīn	loss of voice
气促	qì-cù	panting
骨蒸	gǔ-zhēng	steaming bones
盗汗	dào-hàn	thief sweating
面色	miàn-sè	facial color; complexion

皓白	hào-bái	shiny white
顴	quán	cheek
妆	zhuāng	make-up; rouge
甚	shèn	severe

Translation 7.5

4. Worms: Roundworm, pinworm, and tapeworm are commonly seen intestinal parasites. Often they are generated because of a permanent dominance of dampness and heat, because drink or food were unclean, or following a consumption of raw vegetables, gourds, or fruit, and fragrant, dry, fat, and sweet (things) simultaneously. The pathoconditions accompanying a suffering from an intestinal parasite illness manifest themselves as yellow face with emaciated flesh, a black color in the eye socket and below the nose, itching in the nostrils and in the anus, as well as white dots growing inside the lips and resembling millet grains; the appetite decreases, or increases extraordinarily. Some (patients) long to eat raw rice, or tea leaves. Pains of birth (develop) in the abdomen, and the face changes its color. In children (intestinal parasites) especially easily cause malnutrition accumulations; the abdomen grows big, hardens, and (develops a feeling of) fullness. This is commonly called malnutrition inflation/food accumulation. Consumption, that is (the formerly so-called) corpse transmitted consumption, is transmitted by consumption worms. The illness sits in the lung. Coughing and haemoptysis, loss of voice and panting, steaming bones[1] and thief sweating,[2] shiny white complexion, and cheeks as if painted with rouge appear as pathoconditions. The harm to a person is very severe.

Notes

1 The notion of "steaming bones" originated in traditional chinese pediatrics. It is based on an assumption that periodically appearing fevers were normal phenomena whereby surplus heat is effused through the bones in the natural course of a child's development.

2 The term "thief-sweating" denotes nocturnal sweating. This condition happens unbeknown to a patient during sleep like the surreptitious entry of a thief.

Text 7.6

病因虽分外因和内因，但不能把它们孤立起来看。中医分疾病为外感和内伤两大类，就以六淫和七情作为两者的主因，其实，外因不通过内因不容易侵害人体，同样地内因也往往由外因而引发。同时，除了发病的主因之外，还应当注意其他因素，如生活，营养，居住条件等，均有极大关系。

Transliteration 7.6

Bìng-yīn suī fēn wài-yīn hé nèi-yīn, dàn bù néng bǎ tā-men gū-lì qǐ-lái kàn. Zhōng-yī fēn jí-bìng wéi wài-gǎn hé nèi-shāng liǎng dà lèi, jiù yǐ liù-yín hé qī-qíng zuò-wéi liǎng zhě de zhǔ-yīn, qí-shí, wài-yīn bù tōng-guò nèi-yīn bù róng-yì qīn-hài rén-tǐ, tóng-yàng de nèi-yīn yě wǎng-wǎng yóu wài-yīn ér yǐn-fā. Tóng-shí, chú-le fā-bìng de zhǔ-yīn zhī wài, hái yīng-dāng zhù-yì qí-tā yīn-sù, rú shēng-huó, yíng-yǎng, jū-zhù tiáo-jiàn děng, jūn yǒu jí-dà guān-xi.

Vocabulary 7.6

看	kàn	view
主因	zhǔ-yīn	major cause
其实	qí-shí	in fact
容易	róng-yì	simple
侵害	qīn-hài	enter and cause harm
引发	yǐn-fā	bring forth
其他	qí-tā	others
居住	jū-zhù	reside

Translation 7.6

Although (Chinese medicine) divides the causes of illness into external causes and internal causes, they cannot be looked at separately. Chinese medicine divides the illnesses into the two large categories of external affection and internal harm, and it considers the six excesses and the seven affects as the major causes within these two (categories). The fact is, (though), that the external causes cannot enter the human body and cause harm there if not through (the help of) internal causes; and, similarly, the internal causes often enough emerge only because of external causes. Moreover, attention should be paid not only to the major cause that has brought about an illness, but also to other factors, such as the conditions of (a person's) lifestyle, nourishment, and housing. They all are closely related (to the causation of illness).

Text 7.7

疾病的发生，有意外损害，既不属于内因，又不属于外因，称为不内外因。

1. 房室伤：指色欲过度，精气受伤。不仅身体虚弱，还易招致病邪。

2. 金刃伤：指刀剑创伤或跌打损伤一类。

3. 汤火伤：指汤水烫伤或火灼烧伤。

4. 虫兽伤：指毒蛇猛兽等咬伤，除了体表受到直接伤害外，还能引起不同程度的中毒。

5. 中毒：一般多指食物中毒或药物中毒。

不内外因和内因，外因也有关系，譬如刀伤后外邪再从创口侵入，能发生严重的破伤风症。所以三因中任何一因都不能把它孤立起来。

Transliteration 7.7

Jí-bìng de fā-shēng, yǒu yì-wài sǔn-hài, jí bù shǔ-yú nèi-yīn, yòu bù shǔ-yú wài-yīn, chēng-wéi bù-nèi-wài-yīn.

1. Fáng-shì-shāng: zhǐ sè-yù guò-dù, jīng-qì shòu shāng. Bù-jǐn shēn-tǐ xū-ruò, hái yì zhāo-zhì bìng-xié.

2. Jīn-rèn-shāng: chǐ dāo-jiàn chuāng-shāng huò diē-dǎ sǔn-shāng yī lèi.

3. Tāng-huǒ-shāng: zhǐ tāng-shuǐ tàng-shāng huò huǒ-zhuó-shāo-shāng.

4. Chóng-shòu shāng: zhǐ dú-shé měng-shòu děng yǎo-shāng, chú-le tǐ-biǎo shòu-dào zhí-jiē shāng-hài wài, hái néng yǐn-qǐ bù-tóng chéng-dù de zhòng-dú.

5. Zhòng-dú: yī-bān duō zhǐ shí-wù-zhòng-dú huò yào-wù-zhòng-dú. Bù-nèi-wài-yīn hé nèi-yīn, wài-yīn yě yǒu guān-xi, pì-rú dāo-shāng hòu wài-xié zài cóng chuāng-kǒu qīn-rù, néng fā-shēng yán-zhòng de pò-shāng-fēng zhèng. Suǒ-yǐ sān-yīn zhōng rèn-hé yī yīn, dōu bù néng bǎ tā gū-lì qǐ-lái.

Vocabulary 7.7

意外	yì-wài	accident
损害	sǔn-hài	injury
既不 ... 又不 ...	jì-bù ... yòu-bù ...	neither ... nor ...
房室	fáng-shì	bedroom
房室伤	fáng-shì-shāng	harm from sexual intercourse
色欲	sè-yù	sexual desire
招致	zhāo-zhì	invite
金刃伤	jīn-rèn-shāng	injury from metal blades
刀剑	dāo-jiàn	knives and swords
跌打	diē-dǎ	fall
损伤	sǔn-shāng	injury; injure
汤火伤	tāng-huǒ-shāng	injury from hot liquid and fire
汤水	tāng-shuǐ	hot water
烫伤	tàng-shāng	scalding
火灼烧伤	huǒ-zhuó-shāo-shāng	burn
兽	shòu	quadrupeds; animals
虫兽伤	chóng-shòu shāng	injury from insects and animals
毒蛇	dú-shé	poisonous snake
猛兽	měng-shòu	wild animal
咬伤	yǎo-shāng	injury from a bite
伤害	shāng-hài	harm; damage
程度	chéng-dù	degree
中毒	zhòng-dú	poisoning
食物中毒	shí-wù-zhòng-dú	food poisoning
药物中毒	yào-wù-zhòng-dú	drug poisoning
譬如	pì-rú	for example
刀伤	dāo-shāng	injury from a knife

创口	chuāng-kǒu	opening of a wound
侵入	qīn-rù	invade
破伤风	pò-shāng-fēng	tetanus
三因	sān-yīn	the three causes (of illness)

Translation 7.7

If the emergence of an illness has (its origin in) an accidental injury, then (this injury) neither belongs to the (category of) internal causes, nor does it belong to the eternal causes. It is called a neither-internal-nor-external cause.

1. Harm from sexual intercourse: (This) refers to harm received by (a person's) essence and qi because of sexual excesses. Not only does the body become depleted and weak, it also easily invites an evil that may lead to illness.

2. Injury from weapons: (This) refers to the group of wounds from knives or swords, and of injuries received from accidental falls.

3. Injury from hot liquids and fire: (This) refers to scalding by hot water, and to burns by fire.

4. Injury from insects and animals: (This) refers to bite injuries received from poisonous snakes and wild animals. In addition to direct wounds received at the outside of the body, (such bites) may also evoke poisonings of different degrees.

5. Poisoning: In general (this) refers to food or drug poisoning.

The neither-internal-nor-external causes (of illness) are related to the internal causes and to the external causes. For example, after an injury from a knife, an external evil may enter (the body) through the open wound, and cause a very serious tetanus condition. Hence any of the three causes must not be isolated (from the others).

Text 7.8

病之来，必有因，一个原因可以生出多种不同的病，而同一病症也可由各种不同的原因造成。所以中医有"异病同治，同病异治"的特点，一个药方能治几种不同的病，有时在一种病上又必须用几个药方来治疗。例如同一热邪，有的表现为发热，有的咳嗽，有的失血，只要求得是热邪，病症虽异都能用清凉剂；又如同一发热，有因热邪，因寒邪，因血症而起的，发热虽同而所以引起发热的原因不同，就不能专用清凉剂退热了。这是说明病因对于治疗的重要性，故治疗任何一种病，首先要把原因弄清楚。

Transliteration 7.8

Bìng zhī lái, bì yǒu yīn, yī ge yuán-yīn kě-yǐ shēng-chū duō zhǒng bù-tóng de bìng, ér tóng-yī bìng-zhèng yě kě yóu gè zhǒng bù-tóng de yuán-yīn zào-chéng. Suǒ-yǐ zhōng-yī yǒu "yì bìng tóng zhì, tóng bìng yì zhì" de tè-diǎn, yī ge yào-fāng néng zhì jǐ zhǒng bù-tóng de bìng, yǒu-shí zài yī zhǒng bìng shàng yòu bì-xū yòng jǐ-gè yàofāng lái zhì-liáo. Lì-rú tóng-yī rè-xié, yǒu-de biǎo-xiàn wéi fā-rè, yǒu-de ké-sòu, yǒu-de shī-xuè, zhǐ yào qiú-de shì rè-xié, bìng-zhèng suī yì dōu néng yòng qīng-liáng-jì; yòu-rú tóng-yī fā-rè, yǒu yīn rè-xié, yīn hán-xié, yīn xuè-zhèng ér qǐ de, fā-rè suī tóng ér suǒ-yǐ yǐn-qǐ fā-rè de yuán-yīn bù-tóng, jiù bù néng zhuān yòng qīng-liáng-jì tuì rè le. Zhè shì shuō-míng bìng-yīn duì-yú zhì-liáo de zhòng-yào xìng, gù zhì-liáo rèn-hé yī zhǒng bìng, shǒu-xiān yào bǎ yuán-yīn nòng qīng-chu.

Vocabulary 7.8

原因	yuán-yīn	cause
生出	shēng-chū	generate
同一	tóng-yī	identical
造成	zào-chéng	bring forth
药方	yào-fāng	formula; prescription
几	jǐ	some
几个	jǐ-gè	some
失血	shī-xuè	loss of blood
求得	qiú-de	find out

是	shì	this
清凉剂	qīng-liáng-jì	cooling prescription
又如	yòu-rú	as a further example; on the other hand
血症	xuè-zhèng	blood condition
专	zhuān	only; exclusively
退	tuì	push back
任何	rèn-hé	each; any
首先	shǒu-xiān	first
弄	nòng	make; do
清楚	qīng-chu	clear

Translation 7.8

The onset of an illness must have a cause; one single cause can generate many different illnesses, and one and the same illness can have been brought forth by all kinds of different causes. Hence Chinese medicine has the characteristic of "like treatment of unlike illnesses; unlike treatment of like illnesses." One and the same prescription can treat several different illnesses; sometimes it is necessary to employ several prescriptions to treat identical illnesses. For example, one identical heat evil may manifest itself as fever, or as cough, or as loss of blood. All that is necessary is to find out this heat evil. Even though the pathoconditions are different, in all cases cooling formulas can be employed. On the other hand, identical fevers may have been brought about by a heat evil, or by a cold evil, or because of a blood condition. Even though the fevers are identical, the causes that have brought about these fevers are different. Hence it is inappropriate to use only cooling formulas to decrease the heat. This explains the importance of the causes of an illness in view of a therapy. Hence for the treatment of any illness, (its) causes must be clarified first of all.

Text 8.1

每一个病，都有错综复杂的症状，要找到它的关键，掌握它的主要方面，必须懂得运用八纲。八纲就是阴阳，表里，寒热，虚实，为辨症的纲领，其中阴阳尤为纲领的纲领。表里，寒热，虚实，实际上是阴阳的演绎，亦称六变，它指示了病变所在的部位，病情的征象和邪正消长的变化。所以根据八纲来观察症候的全部情况，加以分析归纳，不难得出诊断结论。关于阴阳方面已在

第一章叙述，兹再就六变的意义，说明如下。

Transliteration 8.1

Měi-yī-ge bìng, dōu yǒu cuò-zōng-fù-zá de zhèng-zhuàng, yào zhǎo-dào tā-de guān-jiàn, zhǎng-wò tā-de zhǔ-yào fāng-miàn, bì-xū dǒng-de yùn-yòng bā-gāng. Bā-gāng jiù-shì yīn yáng, biǎo lǐ, hán rè, xū shí, wéi biàn-zhèng de gāng-lǐng, qí-zhōng yīn yáng yóu wéi gāng-lǐng de gāng-lǐng. Biǎo lǐ, hán rè, xū shí, shí-jì-shàng shì yīn yáng de yǎn-yì, yì chēng liù-biàn, tā zhǐ-shì le bìng-biàn suǒ zài de bù-wèi, bìng-qíng de zhēng-xiàng hé xié zhèng xiāo-zhǎng de biàn-huà. Suǒ-yǐ gēn-jù bā-gāng lái guān-chá zhèng-hòu de quán-bù qíng-kuàng, jiā-yǐ fēn-xī guī-nà, bù nán dé-chū zhěn-duàn jié-lùn. Guān-yú yīn yáng fāng-miàn yǐ zài dì yī zhāng xù-shù, zī zài jiù liù-biàn de yì-yì, shuō-míng rú xià.

Vocabulary 8.1

每一个	měi-yī-gè	each
错综复杂	cuò-zōng-fù-zá	complex
找到	zhǎo-dào	find out
关键	guān-jiàn	key point
掌握	zhǎng-wò	grasp
懂得	dǒng-de	understand
八纲	bā-gāng	the eight principles
辨症	biàn-zhèng	the differentiation of the pathoconditions
纲领	gāng-lǐng	guiding principle
演绎	yǎn-yì	deduct
实际上	shí-jì-shàng	in reality
六变	liù-biàn	the six changes

指示	zhǐ-shì	refer to
征象	zhēng-xiàng	sign
正	zhèng	proper; correct; right
消长	xiāo-zhǎng	waning and waxing
全部	quán-bù	entirety
加以	jiā-yǐ	amend by; add
得出	dé-chū	get
结论	jié-lùn	conclusion
关于	guān-yú	as regards
第	dì	(particle indicating that the following number is an ordinal number)
章	zhāng	chapter
叙述	xù-shù	discuss; outline
兹	zī	here; now

Translation 8.1

Each illness is accompanied by complex pathoconditions; if (someone) wishes to find out its key points, and if (that person wishes) to grasp its major aspects, (he/she) must understand how to employ the eight principles. The eight principles are yin and yang, outside and inside, cold and heat, and depletion as well as repletion. They constitute the guiding principles in the differentiation of the pathoconditions. Among them, yin and yang in particular represent the guiding principles of the (other) guiding principles. Outside and inside, cold and heat, as well as depletion and repletion are, in fact, deductions of yin and yang; they are also called the six changes. They refer to the locations where pathological changes take place, to the appearances of the illnesses, and to the changes in the waxing and waning of evil and proper (qi). Hence, if the circumstances of the pathological signs (of an illness) are examined in their entirety on the basis of the eight principles, and if analytical, deductive considerations are added, it will not be difficult to reach a diagnostic conclusion. Yin and yang have been discussed in chapter one already; here, in addition, only the meaning of the six changes is explained as follows.

Text 8.2

1. 表里：表是外，里是内。从人体的内外来说，表是体表，包括皮肤，肌肉等组织；里是指内脏，包括脏，腑和脑等器官。因此病邪侵犯人体所出现的症状，如恶寒，发热，头痛，项强，身疼，四肢酸软，以及有汗，无汗等症，属于体表者均为表症；神昏烦躁，口渴胸闷，呕吐泄泻，腹痛腹胀等症，属于体内者，均为里症。

Transliteration 8.2

1. Biǎo lǐ: biǎo shì wài, lǐ shì nèi. Cóng rén-tǐ de nèi-wài lái shuō, biǎo shì tǐ-biǎo, bāo-kuò pí-fū, jī-ròu děng zǔ-zhī; lǐ shì zhǐ nèi-zàng, bāo-kuò zàng, fǔ hé nǎo děng qì-guān. Yīn-cǐ bìng-xié qīn-fàn rén-tǐ suǒ chū-xiàn de

zhèng-zhuàng, rú wù-hán, fā-rè, tóu-tòng, xiàng-jiàng, shēn-téng, sì-zhī suān-ruǎn, yǐ-jí yǒu hàn, wú-hàn děng, zhèng shǔ-yú tǐ-biǎo zhě jūn wéi biǎo-zhèng; shén-hūn fán-zào, kǒu-kě xiōng-mèn, ǒu-tù xiè-xiè, fù-tòng fù-zhàng děng, zhèng shǔ-yú tǐ-nèi zhě jūn wéi lǐ-zhèng.

Vocabulary 8.2

肌肉	jī-ròu	muscles
器官	qì-guān	organ
项强	xiàng-jiàng	stiff neck
身疼	shēn-téng	body pains
酸软	suān-ruǎn	painful and weak
无汗	wú-hàn	absence of sweating
腹胀	fù-zhàng	abdominal swelling

Translation 8.2

1. Outside and inside: outside is the outer; inside is the inner. In terms of the outer and inner of the human body, the "outside" is the outside of the body, including tissues such as skin and muscles. "Inside" refers to the inner depots, and includes organs such as the depots, the palaces, and the brain. Hence of the pathoconditions manifesting themselves when an illness evil has entered the human body, pathoconditions such as aversion to cold, fever, headache, stiff neck, body pains, aching limbs, as well as sweat or absence of sweat, belong to the body's outside and are all alike outside pathoconditions. Pathoconditions such as mental confusion and restlessness, thirst and a feeling of pressure in the chest, vomiting and diarrhea, abdominal pain and abdominal swelling, belong to the inner (section) of the body, and are all inside pathoconditions.

Text 8.3

风，寒等六淫之邪侵犯人体，首先伤于皮毛，经络，概称表症。因喜怒七情或饮食劳倦所引起的病，多自内生，故概称里症。这是辨别表里的概况。但表邪可以内传进入脏腑，则其所现的症状又为里症了。也有表邪虽已内传而尚未到里，称为半表半里症。表邪内传而表症仍在，称为表里同病。因此，临症上分辨表里症，更重要的是注意其传变倾向。

Transliteration 8.3

Fēng, hán děng liù-yín zhī xié qīn-fàn rén-tǐ, shǒu-xiān shāng yú pí máo, jīng-luò, gài chēng biǎo-zhèng. Yīn xǐ nù qī-qíng huò yǐn-shí láo-juàn suǒ yǐn-qǐ de bìng, duō zì nèi shēng, gù gài chēng lǐ-zhèng. Zhè shì biàn-bié biǎo lǐ de gài-kuàng. Dàn biǎo-xié kě-yǐ nèi chuán jìn-rù zàng-fǔ, zé qí suǒ xiàn de zhèng-zhuàng yòu wéi lǐ-zhèng le. Yě yǒu biǎo-xié suī yǐ nèi chuán ér shàng wèi dào lǐ, chēng-wéi bàn-biǎo-bàn-lǐ-zhèng. Biǎo-xié nèi chuán ér biǎo-zhèng réng zài, chēng-wéi biǎo-lǐ-tóng-bìng. Yīn-cǐ, lín-zhèng shàng fēn-biàn biǎo lǐ zhèng, gèng zhòng-yào de shì zhù-yì qí chuán-biàn qīng-xiàng.

Vocabulary 8.3

概	gài	in general; summarily
劳倦	láo-juàn	weariness from toil
辨别	biàn-bié	distinguish
概况	gài-kuàng	rough survey
表邪	biǎo-xié	outside evil
传	chuán	transmit; be transmitted
进入	jìn-rù	enter
半表半里症	bàn-biǎo-bàn-lǐ-zhèng	half-outside-half-inside pathocondition
仍	réng	still
表里同病	biǎo-lǐ-tóng-bìng	joint illness outside and inside
分辨	fēn-biàn	differentiate

Translation 8.3

When an evil of any of the six excesses, such as wind or cold, invades the human body, it will cause harm first to the skin and its hair, and to the conduits and network (vessels). (The resulting pathoconditions) are summarily called outside pathoconditions. Illnesses that have been brought forth by the seven affects, such as joy or anger, or by food and drink, and weariness from toil, emerge mostly from the interior; hence they are summarily called inside pathoconditions. This is a rough survey how to distinguish between outside and inside. However, outside evils can be transmitted to the interior, and enter the depots and palaces, and the pathoconditions which appear are inside pathoconditions too. It may also be that an outside evil has been transmitted to the interior already but has not yet reached the inside. This is called a half-outside-half-inside pathocondition. If an outside evil has been transmitted to the interior with the outside pathoconditions present nevertheless, this is called joint illness outside and inside. Hence in the differentiation between outside and inside pathoconditions in clinical practice, it is even more important (than to merely differentiate between outside and inside) to pay attention to the directions of their transmissions and change.

2. 寒热：寒的症状为口不作渴，喜饮热汤，手足厥冷，无风恶寒，小便清长，大便溏薄，面色苍白，舌苔白滑，脉迟。热的症状为口渴饮凉，潮热，烦躁，小便短黄，大便闭结，面红目赤，舌苔黄糙，脉数等。这里可以看出病情的表现有寒和热两种不同的现象，辨别寒，热，就是决定用药或温或凉的一个关键。寒症和热症有时不完全是全身症状，如发热是全身的，小溲黄赤可以与发热有关，也有仅属于膀胱有热。所以辨寒症和热症除一般者外，需要进一步分别上下。

Transliteration 8.4

2. Hán rè: hán de zhèng-zhuàng wéi kǒu-bù-zuò-kě, xǐ yǐn rè tāng, shǒu zú jué-lěng, wú fēng wù-hán, xiǎo-biàn qīng cháng, dà-biàn táng-bó, miàn-sè cāng-bái, shé-tāi bái-huá, mài chí. Rè de zhèng-zhuàng wéi kǒu-kě yǐn liáng, cháo-rè, fán-zào, xiǎo-biàn duǎn huáng, dà-biàn bì-jié, miàn hóng mù-chì, shé-tāi huáng cāo, mài shuò děng. Zhè-lǐ kě-yǐ kàn-chū bìng-qíng de biǎo-xiàn yǒu hán hé rè liǎng zhǒng bù-tóng de xiàn-xiàng, biàn-bié hán, rè, jiù-shì jué-dìng yòng-yào huò wēn huò liáng de yī ge guān-jiàn. Hán-zhèng hé rè-zhèng yǒu-shí bù wán-quán shì quán-shēn zhèng-zhuàng, rú fā-rè shì quán-shēn de, xiǎo-sōu huáng chì kě-yǐ yǔ fā-rè yǒu-guān, yě yǒu jǐn shǔ-yú páng-guāng yǒu rè. Suǒ-yǐ biàn hán-zhèng hé rè-zhèng chú yī-bān zhě wài, xū-yào jìn-yī-bù fēn-bié shàng xià.

Vocabulary 8.4

口不作渴	kǒu-bù-zuò-kě	lack of thirst
汤	tāng	hot liquid
厥冷	jué-lěng	recession (of yang qi giving rise to) cold
苍白	cāng-bái	greenish white
白滑	bái-huá	white glossy
潮	cháo	wave
潮热	cháo-rè	tidal fever
这里	zhè-lǐ	here
完全	wán-quán	complete
小溲	xiǎo-sōu	urinate; urine

仅	jǐn	only; merely
除 ... 外	chú ... wài	except for ...

Translation 8.4

2. Cold and Heat: Pathological manifestations (in case) of (harm caused by) cold are lack of thirst, a desire to drink hot liquids, recession (of yang qi giving rise to) cold in hands and feet, aversion to cold in the absence of wind, clear and extended urination, semiliquid stools, greenish white facial complexion, white glossy tongue coating, and a retarded pulse. Pathoconditions resulting from heat are thirst (with the desire) to drink cold (beverages), tidal fevers, irritability and restlessness, short voidings of yellow urine, constipation, red face and red eyes, rough yellow tongue coating, and a frequent pulse. The manifestations of the nature of the illnesses that can be observed here are the two different appearances of (the underlying illnesses of) cold and heat. The differentiation between cold and heat is a key element in deciding about the use of drugs, whether (to employ) warming or cooling (formulas). Sometimes pathoconditions resulting from cold and pathoconditions of heat are not necessarily pathological manifestations involving the entire body. For example, fever is (a pathocondition) involving the entire body. Yellow or reddish urine may be related to (such) a fever (involving the entire body, but) it may also be that it is related merely to heat in the bladder. Hence in addition to a general differentiation between pathoconditions of cold and those of heat, it is necessary to go a step further and distinguish whether (such a pathocondition) is located in the upper or lower (sections of the body).

3. 虚实：虚实是指正气和邪气两方面来说的。从人体说，指正气的强弱；从病情说，指邪气的盛衰。但在一般临症上，虚多指正气，实多指邪气，因正气充旺无所谓实，邪气退却无所谓虚。虚症的表现，为神疲乏力，声音低怯，呼吸气短，自汗盗汗，头晕心悸，脉细微弱。实症的表现，为痰多气壅，胸闷腹胀，便闭或溏薄臭秽，脉洪滑大等。凡体壮新病，症多属实，体弱久病，症多属虚。患者体质和病理机转表现为有余，结实，强盛的，称为实症；反之，表现为不足，衰退，松弛的，称为虚症。

Transliteration 8.5

3. Xū shí: xū shí shì zhǐ zhèng-qì hé xié-qì liǎng fāng-miàn lái shuō de. Cóng rén-tǐ shuō, zhǐ zhèng-qì de qiáng-ruò; cóng bìng-qíng shuō, zhǐ xié-qì de shèng-shuāi. Dàn zài yī-bān lín-zhèng shàng, xū duō zhǐ zhèng-qì, shí duō zhǐ xié-qì, yīn zhèng-qì chōng wàng wú suǒ wèi shí, xié-qì tuì-què wú suǒ-wèi xū. Xū-zhèng de biǎo-xiàn, wéi shén-pí fá-lì, shēng-yīn dī-qiè, hū-xī qì-duǎn, zì-hàn dào-hàn, tóu-yūn xīn-jì, mài xì wēi ruò. Shí-zhèng de biǎo-xiàn, wéi tán duō qì-yōng, xiōng-mèn fù-zhàng, biàn-bì huò táng-bó chòu-huì, mài hóng huá dà děng. Fán tǐ zhuàng xīn bìng, zhèng duō shǔ shí, tǐ ruò jiǔ bìng, zhèng duō shǔ xū. Huàn zhě tǐ-zhì hé bìng-lǐ jī-zhuǎn biǎo-xiàn wéi yǒu-yú, jiē-shí, qiáng-shèng de, chēng-wéi shí-zhèng; fǎn-zhī, biǎo-xiàn wéi bù-zú, shuāi-tuì, sōng-chí de, chēng-wéi xū-zhèng.

Vocabulary 8.5

A是指B来说的	A shì zhǐ B lái shuō de	lit. "A is spoken (i.e., used) to point (i.e., refer) to B;" A refer(s) to B
从A来说	cóng A lái shuo	lit: "from (the point of view of) A;" as far as A is concerned
盛衰	shèng-shuāi	flourishing and frailty
无所谓 ...	wú suǒ wèi ...	it is impossible to speak of ...
退却	tuì-què	abate

神疲	shén-pí	mental weakness
乏力	fá-lì	lack of physical strength
声音	shēng-yīn	voice
呼吸	hū-xī	breath
气短	qì-duǎn	shortness of breath
头晕	tóu-yūn	dizziness
细	xì	fine
实症	shí-zhèng	pathocondition of repletion
臭秽	chòu-huì	foul
壮	zhuàng	strong
新	xīn	new; just
久	jiǔ	long; chronic
机转	jī-zhuǎn	process
结实	jiē-shí	firm; strong; stable
强盛	qiáng-shèng	strength and abundance
反之	fǎn-zhī	in contrast
松弛	sōng-chí	slacken

Translation 8.5

3. Depletion and Repletion: Depletion and repletion refer to the two (opposite) aspects proper qi and evil qi. In view of the human body, they refer to the strength and weakness of the proper qi. In view of illnesses, they refer to the flourishing and frailty of evil qi. However, in general clinical practice, depletion often refers to proper qi, (while) repletion often refers to evil qi. The reason is, it is impossible to speak of repletion when the proper qi abounds, and it is impossible to speak of depletion when evil qi has abated. Manifestations of pathoconditions of depletion are mental weakness and lack of physical strength, a low and timid voice, shortness of breath, spontaneous sweating and night sweat, dizziness and palpitations, as well as a fine, faint, and weak pulse. Manifestations of pathoconditions of repletion are abundance of phlegm and qi blockages, a feeling of pressure in the chest and abdominal swellings, constipation or semiliquid and foul stools, as well as a vast, smooth, and strong pulse.

Whenever someone with a strong body has just fallen ill, (his/her) pathoconditions mostly belong to (the category of) repletion; the pathoconditions of (people with) weak bodies and chronic illnesses often belong to (the category of) depletion. When the appearances of the patient's physical constitution and of the pathological processes are those of surplus, stability, strength, and abundance, they are called pathoconditions of repletion. In contrast, when the manifestations are those of insufficiency, weakness, and recession or slackening, they are called pathoconditions of depletion.

Text 8.6

辨别虚实是攻邪和补正的根据。病有纯虚纯实者，辨别较易，治疗亦简单；有虚实错杂者，如正强邪实虽重能挽救，正虚邪实虽轻亦危殆。在每一个病的过程中，经常出现邪正消长现象，必须注意虚中有实，实中有虚，虚多实少，虚少实多等变化情况。例如外感风寒，恶寒发热，脉象浮紧，这是一个表实症；如果发汗后汗出不止，身热骤降，反而畏冷更剧，这是转为虚症的症象；或者恶寒退却，身热增加，口渴引饮，这是转为里症的症象。

Transliteration 8.6

Biàn-bié xū shí shì gōng xié hé bǔ zhèng de gēn-jù. Bìng yǒu chún-xū chún-shí zhě, biàn-bié jiào yì, zhì-liáo yì jiǎn-dān; yǒu xū shí cuò-zá zhě, rú zhèng qiáng xié shí suī zhòng néng wǎn-jiù, zhèng xū xié shí suī qīng yì wēi-dài. Zài měi-yī-ge bìng de guò-chéng zhōng, jīng-cháng chū-xiàn xié zhèng xiāo-zhǎng xiàn-xiàng, bì-xū zhù-yì xū zhōng yǒu shí, shí zhōng yǒu xū, xū duō shí shǎo, xū shǎo shí duō děng biàn-huà qíng-kuàng. Lì-rú wài-gǎn fēng-hán, wù-hán fā-rè, mài-xiàng fú jǐn, zhè shì yī ge biǎo-shí-zhèng; rú-guǒ fā-hàn hòu hàn-chū bù-zhǐ, shēn-rè zhòu jiàng, fǎn ér wèi lěng gèng jù, zhè shì zhuǎn-wéi xū-zhèng de zhèng-xiàng; huò zhě wù-hán tuì-què, shēn-rè zēng-jiā, kǒu-kě yǐn yǐn, zhè shì zhuǎn-wéi lǐ-zhèng de zhèng-xiàng.

Vocabulary 8.6

攻	gōng	attack
纯虚	chún-xū	pure depletion
纯实	chún-shí	pure repletion
简单	jiǎn-dān	simple
错杂	cuò-zá	mixed
挽救	wǎn-jiù	rescue
亦	yì	still
危殆	wēi-dài	dangerous
经常	jīng-cháng	often
表实症	biǎo-shí-zhèng	pathocondition of outside repletion

发汗	fā-hàn	develop sweat
不止	bù-zhǐ	incessantly
骤	zhòu	dramatically; suddenly
畏	wèi	fear
剧	jù	worsen
转为	zhuǎn-wéi	change into
症象	zhèng-xiàng	sign
增加	zēng-jiā	increase
引	yǐn	draw

Translation 8.6

To differentiate depletion and repletion is the basis of attacking evil and of supplementing proper (qi). To differentiate whether an illness consists of pure depletion or pure repletion, that is relatively easy, and the therapy (of such conditions) is simple too. When depletion and repletion are present simultaneously, even a serious repletion with evil (qi) can be rescued if the proper (qi) is strong, and even a light repletion with evil (qi) may be dangerous if the proper (qi) is depleted. In the course of each illness it is common that a phenomenon of waxing and waning of evil and proper (qi) occurs, and it necessary to pay attention to the (various possible) states of such changes, as are repletion within depletion, depletion within repletion, more depletion and less repletion, and more repletion and less depletion. For example, if someone was affected by wind-cold externally, has an aversion to cold and develops fever, and if (this person's) pulse is at the surface and tight, this is a pathocondition of outside repletion. If after diaphoresis (the patient) sweats incessantly, if the body heat drops all of a sudden and, in contrast, it is to be feared that the cooling down (of the body) even worsens, then these are signs that (the former condition) has changed into a pathocondition of depletion. Sometimes the aversion to cold abates, and the body heat increases. (The patient) is thirsty and drinks. These are signs that (the former condition) has changed into an inside pathocondition.

Text 8.7

表里，寒热，虚实，是一种症状的归纳方法，单看一个症状是没有意思的。因为每一个症状都能在两方面出现，譬如表症有怕冷，里症也有怕冷，虚症有怕冷，实症也有怕冷，寒症有怕冷，热症同样有怕冷。究竟属于哪一类型呢？必须结合多种症状来决定。所以把许多症状加以分析，就其性质上的类同联系起来，成为一个症候群，才能诊断它是表是里，是虚是实，是寒是热。这就说明了辨症的目的是在求得病的本质，要掌握真相，必须从多方面观察。

Transliteration 8.7

Biǎo lǐ, hán rè, xū shí, shì yī zhǒng zhèng-zhuàng de guī-nà fāng-fǎ, dān kàn yī ge zhèng-zhuàng shì méi-yǒu-yì-si-de. Yīn-wéi měi-yī-ge zhèng-zhuàng dōu néng zài liǎng fāng-miàn chū-xiàn, pì-rú biǎo-zhèng yǒu pà-lěng, lǐ-zhèng yě yǒu pà-lěng, xū-zhèng yǒu pà-lěng, shí-zhèng yě yǒu pà-lěng, hán-zhèng yǒu pà-lěng, rè-zhèng tóng-yàng yǒu pà-lěng. Jiū-jìng shǔ-yú nǎ-yī lèi-xíng ne? Bì-xū jié-hé duō zhǒng zhèng-zhuàng lái jué-dìng. Suǒ-yǐ bǎ xǔ-duō zhèng-zhuàng jiā-yǐ fēn-xī, jiù qí xìng-zhì shàng-de lèi tóng lián-xì qǐ-lái, chéng-wéi yī ge zhèng-hòu qún, cái néng zhěn-duàn tā shì biǎo shì lǐ, shì xū shì shí, shì hán shì rè. Zhè jiù shuō-míng le biàn-zhèng de mù-dì shì zài qiú-de bìng de běn-zhì, yào zhǎng-wò zhēn-xiàng, bì-xū cóng duō fāng-miàn guān-chá.

Vocabulary 8.7

没有意思的	méi-yǒu-yì-si-de	meaningless
究竟	jiū-jìng	in the end; finally
哪一	nǎ-yī	which
呢	ne	(particle indicating a question that comes in the natural progression of discourse: "so, ..."?) here: which?
决定	jué-dìng	decide
许多	xǔ-duō	many
把 A 加以 B	bǎ A jiā yǐ B	(structure indicating that A is an object of B)

群	qún	group
目的	mù-dì	goal
本质	běn-zhì	basic nature
真相	zhēn-xiàng	the real facts

Translation 8.7

(The differentiation of) outside and inside, cold and heat, as well as depletion and repletion is a method to classify pathological manifestations. However, it makes no sense to observe only one pathological manifestation. The reason is that each pathological manifestation can manifest itself in two respects. For instance, the pathoconditions of (illnesses in the) outside include aversion to cold, and the pathoconditions of (illnesses in the) inside include an aversion to cold too. The pathoconditions of depletion include an aversion to cold, and the pathoconditions of repletion include an aversion to cold too. The pathoconditions of cold include an aversion to cold, and the pathoconditions of heat equally include an aversion to cold. In the end, then, to which type (of pathocondition) does (aversion to cold) belong? It is essential to combine many pathological manifestations to arrive at a decision. Hence (a therapist) analyses many pathological manifestations, combines those of a similar nature, forms a group of (related) pathological signs, and only then is able to diagnose whether (the problem) is outside or inside, whether it is a depletion or repletion, or whether it is a cold or a heat. This is just to point out that the goal of differentiating pathoconditions is to search for the basic nature of an illness, and if (a therapist) wishes to grasp the real facts, (he/she) must examine (a problem) from many sides.

Text 8.8

八纲辨症的内容，包括了体表和体内的关系，指出了病症的性质和发展情况。辨症的最后阶段是为了治疗，分辨表里可以定出或汗或下，分辨寒热可以定出或温或凉，分辨虚实可以定出或补或泻。但是汗法有辛温发汗，有辛凉发汗；下法也有凉下，温下，其它温法，凉法，补法，泻法，也都有不同的用法。如何来确定具体的治疗方针，非把表里，寒热，虚实结合不可。

Transliteration 8.8

Bā-gāng biàn-zhèng de nèi-róng, bāo-kuò le tǐ-biǎo hé tǐ-nèi de guān-xi, zhǐ chū le bìng-zhèng de xìng-zhì hé fā-zhǎn qíng-kuàng. Biàn-zhèng de zuì-hòu jiē-duàn shì wèi-le zhì-liáo, fēn-biàn biǎo lǐ kě-yǐ dìng-chū huò hàn huò xià, fēn-biàn hán rè kě-yǐ dìng-chū huò wēn huò liáng, fēn-biàn xū shí kě-yǐ dìng-chū huò bǔ huò xiè. Dàn-shì hàn-fǎ yǒu xīn wēn fā-hàn, yǒu xīn liáng fā-hàn; xià-fǎ yě yǒu liáng-xià, wēn-xià, qí-tā wēn-fǎ, liáng-fǎ, bǔ-fǎ, xiè-fǎ, yě dōu yǒu bù-tóng de yòng-fǎ. Rú-hé lái què-dìng jù-tǐ de zhì-liáo fāng-zhēn, fēi bǎ biǎo lǐ, hán rè, xū shí jié-hé bù-kě.

Vocabulary 8.8

内容	nèi-róng	content
发展	fā-zhǎn	development
为了	wèi-le	for; on behalf of
定出	dìng-chū	decide
补法	bǔ-fǎ	method of supplementing
泻法	xiè-fǎ	method of draining
凉下	liáng-xià	cooling purging
温下	wēn-xià	warming purging
用法	yòng-fǎ	application
如何(来)	rú-hé (lái)	how to
确定	què-dìng	decision; decide
具体	jù-tǐ	concrete; specific
方针	fāng-zhēn	approach
非 ... 不可	fēi ... bù-kě	impossible if not ...

Translation 8.8

The contents of (the doctrine of) eight principle pathocondition differentiation (as outlined above) comprise the relationships between the outside and the inside of the body, and they refer to the nature of the illnesses and to the circumstances of their development. The final phase in the differentiation of pathoconditions aims at therapy. To distinguish between outside and inside allows one to decide whether to induce sweating or purging; to distinguish between cold and heat allows one to decide whether to warm or to cool; and to distinguish between depletion and repletion allows one to decide whether to supplement or to drain. However, the pattern of diaphoresis includes diaphoresis with acrid and warming (substances), and diaphoresis with acrid and cooling (substances). The method of draining includes cooling purging and warming purging. All the other patterns of warming, of cooling, of supplementing, and of draining include different patterns of application too. The decision in favor of a specific therapeutic approach is impossible if it is not combined with (a consideration of) outside and inside, cold and heat, as well as depletion and repletion.

Text 9.1

六经的意义，是把人体分作六个区域，在这六个区域内出现的症候作为六个类型。这方法最早见于内经，到伤寒论更细致地作出了有系统的分析和归纳。六经的名称为太阳，阳明，少阳，称作三阳；太阴，少阴，厥阴，称作三阴。分析归纳症状时，就根据其不同性质，凡呈亢奋现象的列于三阳，呈衰退现象的列入三阴。六经辨症，不但广泛地被用于外感病，而且内伤杂症也有很多地方可以引用。

Transliteration 9.1

Liù-jīng de yì-yì, shì bǎ rén-tǐ fēn-zuò liù ge qū-yù, zài zhè liù ge qū-yù nèi chū-xiàn de zhèng-hòu zuò-wéi liù ge lèi-xíng. Zhè fāng-fǎ zuì-zǎo jiàn yú nèi-jīng, dào shāng-hán-lùn gèng xì-zhì de zuò-chū le yǒu xì-tǒng de fēn-xī hé guī-nà. Liù-jīng de míng-chēng wéi tài-yáng, yáng-míng, shào-yáng, chēng-zuò sān-yáng; tài-yīn, shào-yīn, jué-yīn, chēng-zuò sān-yīn. Fēn-xī guī-nà zhèng-zhuàng shí, jiù gēn-jù qí bù-tóng xìng-zhì, fán chéng kàng-fèn xiàn-xiàng de liè-yú sān-yáng, chéng shuāi-tuì xiàn-xiàng de liè-rù sān-yīn. Liù-jīng biàn-zhèng, bù-dàn guǎng-fàn de bèi-yòng yú wài-gǎn-bìng, ér-qiě nèi-shāng zá zhèng yě yǒu hěn duō dì-fāng kě-yǐ yǐn-yòng.

Vocabulary 9.1

六经	liù-jīng	the six conduits
区域	qū-yù	region
最早	zuì-zǎo	earliest
内经	nèi-jīng	(book title; abbreviation of:) [Huangdi Neijing] "Huang Di's Inner Classic"
伤寒论	shāng-hán-lùn	(book title) "On Harm Caused by Cold"
细致	xì-zhì	detailed; fine
作出	zuò-chū	produce; generate
太阳	tài-yáng	major yang
阳明	yáng-míng	yang brilliance
少阳	shào-yáng	minor yang
三阳	sān-yáng	the three yang (conduits)
太阴	tài-yīn	major yin
少阴	shào-yīn	minor yin
厥阴	jué-yīn	ceasing yin
三阴	sān-yīn	the three yin (conduits)
亢奋	kàng-fèn	agitated
列于	liè-yú	assign

列入	liè-rù	assign
被用	bèi-yòng	be used
外感病	wài-gǎn-bìng	illnesses resulting from an external affection
引用	yǐn-yòng	apply; make use of

Translation 9.1

The meaning of the six conduits is to divide the human body into six regions, and to classify the pathoconditions appearing in these six regions into six types. The earliest appearance of this method is in the *Neijing;*[1] by the (time of the) *Shanghan lun*[2] a systematic analysis and classification had been completed in even more detail. The designations of the six conduits are "major yang," "yang brilliance" and "minor yang" – these are called (summarily) the "three yang" – and "major yin," "minor yin" and "ceasing yin" – these are called the three yin. In the analysis and classification of the pathoconditions, on the basis of their different natures all those presenting themselves as excesses are assigned to the three yang, and all those presenting themselves as losses are assigned to the three yin. The differentiation of pathoconditions (according to) the six conduits is not only widely applied in case of illnesses (resulting from) an external affection, it can be applied also in many instances of various pathoconditions resulting from inner harm.

Notes

1 The *Neijing* was compiled, in its major part, during the second and first centuries B.C.. Some of its contents reflect earlier traditions, other parts may have been added as late as during the Tang era. The work as a whole is heterogeneous in content, and deals with theory as well as blood letting and acupuncture, but not with drug therapy. The authors of the individual parts are unknown.

2 The *Shanghan lun* was compiled by Zhang Ji 张机 (Zhongjing 仲景) at the beginning of the third century A.D. It is the first known text to link Chinese pharmaceutics to the yinyang and five phases theories.

Text 9.2

1. 太阳脉症：症见发热恶寒，头项强痛，身疼腰酸，无汗，脉象浮紧。此为寒邪侵表的初期，概称太阳病。太阳病中有自汗，脉浮缓的称中风（即伤风）；伴有口渴而不恶寒，或恶寒轻微的则属温病。

2. 阳明脉症：外邪在太阳经不能及时解除，病邪向里发展。症见壮热，汗多，不恶寒，反恶热，口渴，脉象滑大。此时无形热邪弥漫肠胃，但肠内糟粕尚未成为燥屎，热而未实，称作阳明经症。若肠有燥屎，更见便秘，腹满，腹痛，烦躁谵语，甚至神志昏糊，热而兼实，称作阳明腑症。这是外感的第二期，邪已化火，具有一派热象，故称阳明病。

Transliteration 9.2

1. Tài-yáng-mài zhèng: zhèng jiàn fā-rè wù-hán, tóu xiàng jiáng tòng, shēn-téng yāo-suān, wú-hàn, mài-xiàng fú jǐn. Cǐ wéi hán-xié qīn biǎo de chū-qī, gài chēng tài-yáng-bìng. Tài-yáng-bìng zhōng yǒu zì-hàn, mài fú huǎn de chēng zhòng-fēng (jí shāng-fēng); bàn-yǒu kǒu-kě ér bù wù-hán, huò wù-hán qīng wēi de zé shǔ wēn-bìng.

2.Yáng-míng-mài zhèng: wài-xié zài tài-yáng-jīng bù néng jí-shí jiě-chú, bìng-xié xiàng lǐ fā-zhǎn. Zhèng jiàn zhuàng-rè, hàn duō, bù wù-hán, fǎn wù-rè, kǒu-kě, mài-xiàng huá dà. Cǐ-shí wú-xíng rè-xié mí-màn cháng wèi, dàn cháng nèi zāo-pò shàng wèi chéng-wéi zào-shǐ, rè ér wèi shí, chēng-zuò yáng-míng-jīng zhèng. Ruò cháng yǒu zào-shǐ, gèng jiàn biàn-bì, fù-mǎn, fù-tòng, fán-zào zhān-yǔ, shèn-zhì shén-zhì-hūn-hú, rè ér jiān shí, chēng-zuò yáng-míng-fǔ zhèng. Zhè shì wài-gǎn de dì èr qī, xié yǐ huà huǒ, jù-yǒu yī pài rè-xiàng, gù chēng yáng-míng-bìng.

Vocabulary 9.2

太阳脉	tài-yáng-mài	major yang vessel
侵	qīn	intrude
初期	chū-qī	initial phase
太阳病	tài-yáng-bìng	major yang illness

缓	huǎn	relaxed
伴有	bàn-yǒu	be accompanied by
阳明脉	yáng-míng-mài	yang brilliance vessel
及时	jí-shí	in due time
解除	jiě-chú	remove; eliminate
向	xiàng	towards ...
恶热	wù-rè	aversion to heat
此时	cǐ-shí	at this time
弥漫	mí-màn	penetrate; fill
燥屎	zào-shǐ	dry faeces
若	ruò	if; when
便秘	biàn-bì	constipation
神志昏糊	shén-zhì-hūn-hú	mental confusion
阳明腑	yáng-míng-fǔ	yang brilliance palace
二	èr	two
期	qī	phase
派	pài	group; (measure word)
阳明病	yáng-míng-bìng	yang brilliance illness

Translation 9.2

1. Pathoconditions of the major yang vessels: pathoconditions appearing (here include) fever and an aversion to cold, stiffness and pain in the head and the neck, body pain and soreness of the lumbus, no sweating, and a pulse that is at the surface and tight. These (pathoconditions) represent the initial phase of an intrusion of a cold evil into the (body's) outside; they are summarily called major yang illnesses. If in the course of a major yang illness spontaneous sweating occurs, as well as a pulse that is at the surface and relaxed, this is wind stroke. [This is identical with harm caused by wind]. If (a major yang illness) is accompanied by thirst and if there is no aversion to cold, or if the aversion to cold is insignificant, then it is associated with a warmth illness.

2. Pathoconditions of the yang brilliance vessels: if an external evil in the major yang conduit cannot be eliminated in due time, the illness evil will develop towards the inside. Pathoconditions observed are strong heat, profuse sweating, no aversion to cold, with an aversion to heat instead, thirst, and a pulse that is smooth and strong. At this time a shapeless heat evil penetrates the intestines and the stomach, but the waste in the intestines has not turned into dry faeces. There is heat, but no repletion as yet. These (conditions) are called pathoconditions of the yang brilliance conduit. If there is dry faeces in the intestines, and if there appear, in addition, constipation, abdominal fullness, abdominal pain, vexation and incoherent talk, and in severe cases a mental confusion, then this is heat coupled with repletion. These (conditions) are called pathoconditions of the yang brilliance palace. This is the second phase of an external affection. The evil has turned into fire already, and (the illness) has a heat appearance. Hence it is called yang brilliance illness.

Text 9.3

3. 少阳脉症：病邪从外传内，既不属于太阳表症，又不属于阳明里症，而在太阳阳明的中间阶段。症见寒热往来，一天反复数次，口苦咽干，目眩心烦，呕吐不欲食，脉象弦数。因其处于半表半里之间，故称半表半里症。

4. 太阴脉症：三阳病都有发热症，三阴病以虚症为主，一般没有发热，相反地多呈寒象。太阴病的症状为：腹满自利，或腹痛喜按，口不渴，手足温，呕吐，食不下，脉缓而弱。

Transliteration 9.3

3. Shào-yáng-mài zhèng: bìng-xié cóng wài chuán nèi, jí bù shǔ-yú tài-yáng biǎo-zhèng, yòu bù shǔ-yú yáng-míng lǐ-zhèng, ér zài tài-yáng yáng-míng de zhōng-jiān jiē-duàn. Zhèng jiàn hán rè wǎng-lái, yī tiān fǎn-fù shù-cì, kǒu-kǔ yān-gān, mù-xuàn xīn-fán, ǒu-tù bù yù shí, mài-xiàng xián shuò. Yīn qí chù yú bàn-biǎo-bàn-lǐ zhī-jiān, gù chēng bàn-biǎo-bàn-lǐ-zhèng.

4. Tài-yīn-mài zhèng: sān-yáng-bìng dōu yǒu fā-rè zhèng, sān-yīn-bìng yǐ xū-zhèng wéi zhǔ, yī-bān méi-yǒu fā-rè, xiāng-fǎn de duō chéng hán-xiàng. Tài-yīn-bìng de zhèng-zhuàng wéi: fù-mǎn zì-lì, huò fù-tòng xǐ àn, kǒu bù kě, shǒu zú wēn, ǒu-tù, shí bù xià, mài huǎn ér ruò.

Vocabulary 9.3

少阳脉	shào-yáng-mài	minor yang vessel
中间	zhōng-jiān	be between
往来	wǎng-lái	come and go; pass by
反复	fǎn-fù	return; repeat
数次	shù-cì	several times; repeatedly
目眩	mù-xuàn	dizziness
弦	xián	"string(-like)" (pulse quality)
半表半里	bàn-biǎo-bàn-lǐ	half-outside-half-inside
太阴脉	tài-yīn-mài	major yin vessel
三阳病	sān-yáng-bìng	illnesses of the three yang (conduits)
三阴病	sān-yīn-bìng	illnesses of the three yin (conduits)
太阴病	tài-yīn-bìng	major yin illness
自利	zì-lì	spontaneous discharges

Translation 9.3

3. Pathoconditions of the minor yang vessels: when an illness evil is transmitted from the exterior (body regions) to the interior, it is neither associated with the outside pathoconditions of the major yang, nor is it associated with the inside pathoconditions of the yang brilliance. Rather it is in a phase between the major yang and the yang brilliance. Pathoconditions observed are alternating cold and heat with reversals occurring several times a day, a bitter taste in the mouth and a dry throat, dizziness and vexation, vomiting and no desire to eat, and a pulse that is string(-like) and frequent. Because the location (of the illness evil) is half-way between outside and inside, (its pathoconditions) are called half-outside-half-inside pathoconditions.

4. Pathoconditions of the major yin vessels: all illnesses of the three yang (conduits) are accompanied by pathoconditions of fever. The illnesses of the three yin (conduits) are characterized by depletion, and are usually not accompanied by fever. On the contrary, they often manifest cold phenomena. The pathoconditions of the major yin (vessels) include abdominal fullness and spontaneous discharges, or abdominal pain with pleasure to having (the abdomen) pressed, no thirst, warm hands and feet, vomiting, inability to consume food, and a pulse that is relaxed and weak.

5. 少阴脉症：症见恶寒，四肢厥冷，下利清谷，神疲欲寐，脉象微细。这是阳气虚弱所呈现的全身虚寒症。故少阴病比太阴病更严重一步。但少阴主水火，阳虚则从寒化，阴虚又从火化，因而除上虚寒症外，也有心烦，不得卧及热利，咽痛等内热症出现。

6. 厥阴脉症：厥阴病是外感病的末期，邪正抗争的最后阶段。症状多阴阳错杂，寒症和热症混同呈现，如口渴不止，气上冲胸，心中疼痛觉热，饥不欲食，有时呕出蛔虫。特别是以厥，热交替为特征。厥热交替，即四肢厥冷能自温暖，温暖后又厥冷，厥冷后又温暖。

Transliteration 9.4

5. Shào-yīn-mài zhèng: zhèng jiàn wù-hán, sì-zhī jué-lěng, xià-lì qīng-gǔ, shén-pí yù-mèi, mài-xiàng wēi xì. Zhè shì yáng-qì xū-ruò suǒ chéng-xiàn de quán-shēn xū-hán-zhèng. Gù shào-yīn-bìng bǐ tài-yīn-bìng gèng yán-zhòng yī-bù. Dàn shào-yīn zhǔ shuǐ huǒ, yáng-xū zé cóng hán huà, yīn-xū yòu cóng huǒ huà, yīn-ér chú shàng xū-hán-zhèng wài, yě yǒu xīn-fán, bù dé wò jí rè-lì, yān-tòng děng nèi-rè-zhèng chū-xiàn.

6. Jué-yīn-mài zhèng: jué-yīn-bìng shì wài-gǎn-bìng de mò-qī, xié zhèng kàng-zhēng de zuì-hòu jiē-duàn. Zhèng-zhuàng duō yīn yáng cuò-zá, hán-zhèng hé rè-zhèng hùn-tóng chéng-xiàn, rú kǒu-kě bù-zhǐ, qì shàng chòng xiōng, xīn zhōng téng-tòng jué-rè, jī bù yù shí, yǒu-shí ǒu-chū huí-chóng. Tè-bié shì yǐ jué, rè jiāo-tì wéi tè-zhēng. Jué-rè-jiāo-tì, jí sì-zhī jué-lěng néng zì wēn-nuǎn, wēn-nuǎn hòu yòu jué-lěng, jué-lěng hòu yòu wēn-nuǎn.

Vocabulary 9.4

少阴脉	shào-yīn-mài	minor yin vessel
厥	jué	recede
清谷	qīng-gǔ	undigested food
欲寐	yù-mèi	desire to sleep

虚寒症	xū-hán-zhèng	pathoconditions of depletion cold
少阴病	shào-yīn-bìng	minor yin illness
比	bǐ	in comparison to
更 ... 一步	gèng ... yī-bù	even more ...
热利	rè-lì	heat type diarrhea
咽痛	yān-tòng	pharyngeal pain
内热症	nèi-rè-zhèng	pathoconditions of inner heat
厥阴脉	jué-yīn-mài	ceasing yin vessel
厥阴病	jué-yīn-bìng	ceasing yin illness
末期	mò-qī	final stage
抗争	kàng-zhēng	struggle
混同	hùn-tóng	mixed
冲	chòng	penetrate
觉热	jué-rè	feeling of heat
呕出	ǒu-chū	vomit
交替	jiāo-tì	alternate
厥热交替	jué-rè-jiāo-tì	alternate occurrence of recession (of yang qi) and heat
特征	tè-zhēng	characteristic
温暖	wēn-nuǎn	become warm

Translation 9.4

5. Pathoconditions of the minor yin vessels: pathoconditions observed are aversion to cold, recession (of yang qi causing) cold in the four limbs, diarrhea of undigested food, mental fatigue with a desire to sleep, a pulse quality that is slight and fine. These are pathoconditions of depletion-cold affecting the entire body which appear as a result of yang qi depletion and weakness. Minor yin illnesses are, therefore, even more serious than major yin illnesses. However, the minor yin governs water and fire, and since a yang depletion develops from cold, whereas a yin depletion develops from fire, there appear also in addition to the pathoconditions of depletion cold

(mentioned) above pathoconditions of internal heat such as vexation with inability to rest, as well as heat type diarrhea and pharyngeal pain.

6. Pathoconditions of the ceasing yin vessels: illnesses of the ceasing yin represent the final phase of illnesses contracted from the outside; they are the final stage of the struggle between the evil and the proper. The pathoconditions are often of a mixed yin and yang (type); pathoconditions of cold and pathoconditions of heat appear confused, as for instance unquenchable thirst, rising qi penetrating the chest, pain and a feeling of heat in the heart, hunger with no desire to eat, and an occasional vomiting of roundworms. In particular, the alternate occurrence of recession (of yang qi) and heat is a characteristic feature. In case of an alternate occurrence of recession (of yang qi) and heat, the four limbs affected by recession (of yang qi causing) cold may become warm again spontaneously; after they have become warm they turn cold again with recession (of yang qi). After they have turned cold because of recession (of yang qi), they become warm again.

Text 9.5

六经症状的出现，由于病邪的传变，这种由一经传变到另一经的现象，称作"传经"。传经与否的重要关键，决定于病邪和体力的对比。比如邪气盛，正气弱，传变的机会就多；正气盛，邪气微，传变的机会就少；还有体力强的传变多在三阳，体力衰弱的就容易传到三阴。所以传经不是六经皆传遍，有在太阳不传的，有仅传及阳明，也有传完三阳就痊愈的。

Transliteration 9.5

Liù-jīng zhèng-zhuàng de chū-xiàn, yóu-yú bìng-xié de chuán-biàn, zhè-zhǒng yóu yī jīng chuán-biàn dào lìng-yī jīng de xiàn-xiàng, chēng-zuò "chuán-jīng." Chuán-jīng yǔ-fǒu de zhòng-yào guān-jiàn, jué-dìng yú bìng-xié hé tǐ-lì de duì-bǐ. Bǐ-rú xié-qì shèng, zhèng-qì ruò, chuán-biàn de jī-huì jiù duō; zhèng-qì shèng, xié-qì wēi, chuán-biàn de jī-huì jiù shǎo; hái-yǒu tǐ-lì qiáng de chuán-biàn duō zài sān-yáng, tǐ-lì shuāi-ruò de jiù róng-yì chuán dào sān-yīn. Suǒ-yǐ chuán-jīng bù shì liù-jīng jiē chuán biàn, yǒu zài tài-yáng bù chuán de, yǒu jǐn chuán jí yáng-míng, yě yǒu chuán wán sān-yáng jiù quán-yù de.

Vocabulary 9.5

这种	zhè-zhǒng	this
传经	chuán-jīng	conduit-transmission
否	fǒu	no; not
与否	yǔ-fǒu	or not
对比	duì-bǐ	balance; comparison
正气	zhèng-qì	proper qi
机会	jī-huì	opportunity
遍	biàn	everywhere
完	wán	complete; end
痊愈	quán-yù	cure; heal

Translation 9.5

The appearance of pathoconditions in the six conduits originates from the transmission-transformation of illness evils. The phenomenon of transmission-transformation from one conduit to another is called conduit-transmission. The important key issue whether or not a conduit-transmission will occur is decided by the balance between the illness evil and the strength of the body. If, for example, the evil qi abounds while the proper qi is weak, the opportunities for transmission-transformation are many. If the proper qi abounds while the evil qi is insignificant, then the opportunities for transmission-transformation are few. Also, if the body is strong, transmission-transformations occur mostly in the three yang (conduits), while if the body is weak, (illness evils) are most easily transmitted into the three yin (conduits). Hence a conduit-transmission is not (necessarily) a complete transmission through all six conduits; there are (evils) which are not transmitted in the major yang (conduits), and there are also those (illnesses) that are cured after having been transmitted through the three yang (conduits).

Text 9.6

传经有一定的程序，即按照六经次序由太阳而阳明而少阳而太阴而少阴，终于厥阴，叫做"循经传"。也有不按次序，隔一经或两经相传，如太阳不传阳明而传少阳，或不传少阳而直传阴经，叫做"越经传"。越经传的原因，多由邪盛正虚，病邪乘虚窜入。此外，三阴病有不从阳经传入，一起即见太阴或少阴症状者，称作"直中"。直中的意思是病邪直接侵入，三阴都有直中的病变，但以太阴和少阴为多见。

Transliteration 9.6

Chuán-jīng yǒu yī-dìng de chéng-xù, jí àn-zhào liù-jīng cì-xù yóu tài-yáng ér yáng-míng ér shào-yáng ér tài-yīn ér shào-yīn, zhōng yú jué-yīn, jiào-zuò "xún-jīng-chuán." Yě yǒu bù àn cì-xù, gé yī jīng huò liǎng jīng xiāng-chuán, rú tài-yáng bù chuán yáng-míng ér chuán shào-yáng, huò bù chuán shào-yáng ér zhí chuán yīn-jīng, jiào-zuò "yuè-jīng-chuán." Yuè-jīng-chuán de yuán-yīn, duō yóu xié shèng zhèng xū, bìng-xié chéng xū cuàn-rù. Cǐ-wài, sān-yīn-bìng yǒu bù cóng yáng-jīng chuán-rù, yī qǐ jí jiàn tài-yīn huò shào-yīn zhèng-zhuàng zhě, chēng-zuò "zhí-zhòng." Zhí-zhòng de yì-si shì bìng-xié zhí-jiē qīn-rù, sān-yīn dōu yǒu zhí-zhòng de bìng-biàn, dàn yǐ tài-yīn hé shào-yīn wéi duō jiàn.

Vocabulary 9.6

程序	chéng-xù	sequence; order
终	zhōng	end
循经传	xún-jīng-chuán	transmission following the conduits
越	yuè	skip; bypass
越经传	yuè-jīng-chuán	transmission bypassing (one or two) conduits
窜入	cuàn-rù	enter; invade
传入	chuán-rù	transmit into
一	yī	as soon as
直中	zhí-zhòng	direct strike

Translation 9.6

Conduit-transmissions occur in a definite sequence (of the conduits). That is, when (such a transmission) in accordance with the order of the six conduits starts from the major yang, (continues via) the yang brilliance, the minor yang, the major yin, and the minor yin, and ends in the ceasing yin (conduit), this is called “transmission following the conduits.” There are also transmissions that do not follow this order in that they skip one or two conduits, as for instance when the major yang (conduit) does not transmit (the evil) into the yang brilliance (conduit) but transmits it into the minor yang (conduit), or when it does not transmit it into the minor yang (conduit) but transmits it directly into the yin conduits. That is called transmission bypassing (one or two) conduits. The reason for a transmission bypassing (one or two) conduits lies often in an abundance of evil and a depletion of proper (qi), with the illness evil seizing the depleted (regions) and making quick inroads into (the body). In addition, there are illnesses in the three yin (conduits) that have not been transmitted there from the yang conduits: as soon as they emerge they appear as major yin or minor yin pathoconditions. That is called “direct strike.” The meaning of the term “direct strike” is that the illness evil intrudes directly (into the yin conduits). Pathological changes of direct strike occur in all three yin (conduits), but they appear most often in the major yin and minor yin (conduits).

Text 9.7

六经各有主症主脉，临症上又往往错综出现，例如既有太阳表症，又有阳明里症；或太阳表症还没有完全解除，又出现了阳明里症。前者称作"合病"，后者称作"并病"。它的区别是，合病为两经或三经同时受邪，不是传变所致，遇到这类情况，就称为太阳阳明合病，三阳合病等；并病为一经未退又传一经，必须前一经症状还在，而又具备后一经症状，遇到这类情况，就称为太阳阳明并病，阳明少阳并病等。

Transliteration 9.7

Liù-jīng gè yǒu zhǔ-zhèng zhǔ-mài, lín-zhèng shàng yòu wǎng-wǎng cuò-zōng chū-xiàn, lì-rú jì yǒu tài-yáng biǎo-zhèng, yòu yǒu yáng-míng lǐ-zhèng; huò tài-yáng biǎo-zhèng hái méi-yǒu wán-quán jiě-chú, yòu chū-xiàn le yáng-míng lǐ-zhèng. Qián zhě chēng-zuò "hé-bìng," hòu zhě chēng-zuò "bìng-bìng." Tā-de qū-bié shì, hé-bìng wéi liǎng jīng huò sān jīng tóng-shí shòu xié, bù shì chuán-biàn suǒ-zhì, yù-dào zhè-lèi qíng-kuàng, jiù chēng-wéi tài-yáng yáng-míng hé-bìng, sān-yáng hé-bìng děng; bìng-bìng wéi yī jīng wèi tuì yòu chuán yī jīng, bì-xū qián yī jīng zhèng-zhuàng hái zài, ér yòu jù-bèi hòu yī jīng zhèng-zhuàng, yù-dào zhè-lèi qíng-kuàng, jiù chēng-wéi tài-yáng yáng-míng bìng-bìng, yáng-míng shào-yáng bìng-bìng děng.

Vocabulary 9.7

主症	zhǔ-zhèng	main pathoconditions
主脉	zhǔ-mài	main pulses
既 ... 又 ...	jì ... yòu ...	... as well as ...
合病	hé-bìng	parallel illnesses
并病	bìng-bìng	joint illnesses
这类	zhè-lèi	such
具备	jù-bèi	have

Translation 9.7

Each of the six conduits has its (specific) main pathoconditions and also its (specific) main pulses, but in clinical reality they often appear simultaneously. For instance, there may be present outside pathoconditions of the major yang (conduit), and there may also be present inside pathoconditions of the yang brilliance (conduit). Or, outside pathoconditions of the major yang have not yet been eliminated entirely while inside pathoconditions of the yang brilliance appear in addition. The former (situations) are called "parallel illnesses;" the latter are called "joint illnesses." The difference is that in case of parallel illnesses two or three conduits receive an illness at the same time; (the evil) does not arrive through transmission-transformation. If such a situation is encountered, it is called parallel illnesses of the major yang and yang brilliance, or parallel illnesses of the three yang (conduits). In case of joint illnesses, (the evil) has not left a (particular) conduit yet and was nevertheless transmitted to another conduit already. The pathoconditions of the former conduit must still be present, and in addition the pathoconditions of the second conduit are present too. If such as situation is encountered, it is called (for instance) joint illnesses of the major yang and yang brilliance (conduits), or joint illnesses of the yang brilliance and of the minor yang (conduits).

Text 9.8

用六经来辨症的基本精神已如上述，它不仅说明了外感病发展过程中的一般情况，也说明了六经之间是一个互相影响的整体。这样，可以从全面来观察外感病的发生和变化，从而掌握治疗规律，成为辨症中的一个基本方法。要学习六经辨症，必须对"伤寒论"下一番功夫。"伤寒论"的注解有百数十家，各有特长，比较简明而又能提纲挈领的可阅读尤在泾注的"伤寒贯珠集"，此外，柯韵伯的"伤寒来苏集"

将方证分类，加减变化，眉目朗然，也可作为参考。

Transliteration 9.8

Yòng liù-jīng lái biàn-zhèng de jī-běn jīng-shén yǐ rú shàng-shù, tā bù-jǐn shuō-míng le wài-gǎn-bìng fā-zhǎn guò-chéng zhōng de yī-bān qíng-kuàng, yě shuō-míng le liù-jīng zhī-jiān shì yī ge hù-xiāng yǐng-xiǎng de zhěng-tǐ. Zhè-yàng, kě-yǐ cóng quán-miàn lái guān-chá wài-gǎn-bìng de fā-shēng hé biàn-huà, cóng-ér zhǎng-wò zhì-liáo guī-lǜ, chéng-wéi biàn-zhèng zhōng de yī ge jī-běn fāng-fǎ. Yào xué-xí liù-jīng biàn-zhèng, bì-xū duì "shāng-hán-lùn" xià yī fān gōng-fū. "Shāng-hán-lùn" de zhù-jiě yǒu bǎi-shù-shí-jiā, gè yǒu tè-cháng, bǐ-jiào jiǎn-míng ér yòu néng tí-gāng-qiè-lǐng de kě yuè-dú yóu zài-jīng zhù de "shāng-hán-guàn-zhū-jí," cǐ-wài, kē yùn-bó de "shāng-hán-lái-sū-jí" jiāng fāng zhèng fēn-lèi, jiā-jiǎn biàn-huà, méi-mù lǎng-rán, yě kě zuò-wéi cān-kǎo.

Vocabulary 9.8

全面	quán-miàn	complete; total; entirety
规律	guī-lǜ	law
学习	xué-xí	study
下	xià	apply
番	fān	(measure word for activities)
功夫	gōng-fū	effort; work
对 ... 下一番 功夫	duì ... xià yī fān gōng-fu	make great efforts; devote much time to ...
注解	zhù-jiě	comment
百数十家	bǎi-shù-shí-jiā	many authors
特长	tè-cháng	strength; advantage

比较	bǐ-jiào	relative
简明	jiǎn-míng	simple and clear
提纲挈领	tí-gāng-qiè-lǐng	concentrate on the essential
阅读	yuè-dú	read
尤在泾	yóu zài-jīng	(author's name:) You Zaijing
注	zhù	comment
伤寒贯珠集	shāng-hán-guàn-zhū-jí	(book title:) "Threaded Pearls on Harm caused by Cold"
柯韵伯	kē yùn-bó	(author's name) Ke Yunbo
伤寒来苏集	shāng-hán-lái-sū-jí	(book title:) "Comprehensive Collection on Harm caused by Cold"
方	fāng	prescription
证	zhèng	evidence; sign; (illness) manifestations
分类	fēn-lèi	categorize
加	jiā	add
减	jiǎn	decrease
加减	jiā-jiǎn	increase or decrease; modify
眉目	méi-mù	brows and eyes; headers and titles; logical sequence of thoughts
朗然	lǎng-rán	clear
参考	cān-kǎo	consult

Translation 9.8

The basic spirit of employing the six conduits for differentiating the pathoconditions has been outlined above. It not only illustrates the general conditions of the development processes of illnesses contracted from the outside; it has also shown that the six conduits among each other constitute a unit of mutual influence. This way it is possible to start from the entirety (of the organism), and observe the emergence and transformations of illnesses contracted from the outside, and, thereby, comprehend the laws of treatment (an approach) constituting a basic method in the differentiation of pathoconditions. If someone wishes to study the differentiation of pathoconditions according to the six conduits, (that person) must devote much time to the *Shanghan lun*. Very many authors have written commentaries on the *Shanghan lun,* and each has its particular strengths. As a relatively simple (work) that is nevertheless able to concentrate on the essential, You Zaijing's[1] *Shanghan guanzhuji* can be read. Also, Ke Yunbo's *Shanghan laisuji*[2] is logical and clear in its categorization of prescriptions and (illness) manifestations, and in the (modification of prescriptions) by adding or taking away (substances). It too may serve as consulting (work).

Notes

1 This book was published in 1669.

2 This book was published in 1810.

Text 10.1

中医的诊断方法分为望，闻，问，切，称作四诊。望诊是凭医生的视觉，观察病人的精神，气色，舌苔，及形态和全身各部分情况。

1. 精神：精神的强弱，基于正气的盛衰，正气充实则精神不疲，目光精彩，言语明朗，神思不乱，呼吸平静，虽有临时急症，预后多良。反之，正气衰弱则精神委靡，目光黯淡，言语低怯，神思不定，呼吸气促，虽然临时病势不重，但须防生变端。精神充实的病人，信心高，自主力强，少忧虑，耐痛苦，对疾病能作坚强的斗争，这对治疗是一个有利的条件。

Transliteration 10.1

Zhōng-yī de zhěn-duàn fāng-fǎ fēn-wéi wàng, wén, wèn, qiè, chēng-zuò sì-zhěn. Wàng-zhěn shì píng yī-shēng de shì-jué, guān-chá bìng-rén de jīng-shén, qì-sè, shé-tāi, jí xíng-tài hé quán-shēn gè bù-fèn qíng-kuàng.

1. Jīng-shén: jīng-shén de qiáng-ruò, jī-yú zhèng-qì de shèng-shuāi, zhèng-qì chōng-shí zé jīng-shén bù pí, mù-guāng jīng-cǎi, yán-yǔ míng-lǎng, shén-sī bù-luàn, hū-xī píng-jìng, suī yǒu lín-shí jí-zhèng, yù-hòu duō liáng. Fǎn-zhī, zhèng-qì shuāi-ruò zé jīng-shén wěi-mǐ, mù-guāng àn-dàn, yán-yǔ dī-qiè, shén-sī bù-dìng, hū-xī qì-cù, suī-rán lín-shí bìng-shì bù zhòng, dàn xū fáng shēng biàn-duān. Jīng-shén chōng-shí de bìng-rén, xìn-xīn gāo, zì-zhǔ-lì qiáng, shǎo yōu-lǜ, nài tòng-kǔ, duì jí-bìng néng zuò jiān-qiáng de dòu-zhēng, zhè duì zhì-liáo shì yī ge yǒu-lì de tiáo-jiàn.

Vocabulary 10.1

望	wàng	observe; look
闻	wén	listen; smell
切	qiè	palpate
四诊	sì-zhěn	the four examinations
望诊	wàng-zhěn	visual examination
凭	píng	by means of

医生	yī-shēng	physician
视觉	shì-jué	visual sense
气色	qì-sè	complexion
形态	xíng-tài	the condition of a person's physical appearance
基于	jī-yú	be based on
疲	pí	tired
目光	mù-guāng	eyesight
精彩	jīng-cǎi	brilliant
明朗	míng-lǎng	clear
神思	shén-sī	mental state
不乱	bù-luàn	not in disorder
平静	píng-jìng	quiet
临时	lín-shí	temporarily
急症	jí-zhèng	critical pathocondition
预后	yù-hòu	prognosis
委靡	wěi-mǐ	tired; weak
黯淡	àn-dàn	dim
不定	bù-dìng	unstable
虽然	suī-rán	even though
病势	bìng-shì	the strength of an illness
防	fáng	prevent
变端	biàn-duān	change
信心	xìn-xīn	confidence
高	gāo	high
自主力	zì-zhǔ-lì	power of self-determination
忧虑	yōu-lǜ	worry
痛苦	tòng-kǔ	pain and suffering
坚强	jiān-qiáng	vigorous
斗争	dòu-zhēng	fight
有利	yǒu-lì	beneficial

Translation 10.1

The diagnostic methods of Chinese medicine are classified as looking, listening/smelling, asking, and palpating; (together) they are called the four examinations. A visual examination is to inspect, by means of the physician's visual sense, the patient's essential spirit, complexion, and tongue coating, as well as the condition of his/her physical appearance and of each section of the entire body.

1. The essential spirit: The strength of the essential spirit is based on the abundance of the proper qi; when the proper qi is plentiful, then the essential spirit does not experience fatigue; the eyesight is brilliant, the language is clear, the mental state is not in disorder, and the breathing is quiet. Even if temporarily there may be critical pathoconditions, prognosis is mostly favorable. In contrast, if the proper qi is weak, the spirit is tired, vision is dim, the language is feeble, the mental state is unstable, and the breathing is hasty. Even if the strength of an illness is not serious for the time being, changes (to the worse) are to be prevented. Patients whose essential spirit is substantial have confidence; their power of self-determination is strong, they are rarely worried, they endure pain and suffering, and they are able to put up a vigorous fight against an illness. This is a beneficial factor with respect to their cure.

2.气色：察色包括面部和全身皮肤，分为青，赤，黄，白，黑五种，依据五行学说分属五脏，并将内脏分配在面部各部。比如赤为火之色，主热，就认为肝热病者左颊先赤，肺热病者右颊先赤，心热病者颜先赤，肾热病者颧先赤，脾热病者鼻先赤。这些有其准确的一面，但不能执此一端论定。临症上常见的：面部色青，为小儿急惊，为痰喘重症；青黑为寒痛；色白为气虚，为亡血；色黄为湿气，兼目黄为黄疸；色赤为肝火上逆，为阳明实热，色赤独见两颧者为阴虚火亢；色黑为水气，为女劳疸，妇女眼眶四周色黑者为带下病。

Transliteration 10.2

2. Qì-sè: chá-sè bāo-kuò miàn-bù hé quán-shēn pí-fū, fēn-wéi qīng, chì, huáng, bái, hēi wǔ zhǒng, yī-jù wǔ-xíng xué-shuō fēn-shǔ wǔ-zàng, bìng jiāng nèi-zàng fēn-pèi zài miàn-bù gè bù. Bǐ-rú chì wéi huǒ zhī sè, zhǔ rè, jiù rèn-wéi gān-rè-bìng zhě zuǒ jiá xiān chì, fèi-rè-bìng zhě yòu jiá xiān chì, xīn-rè-bìng zhě yán xiān chì, shèn-rè-bìng zhě quán xiān chì, pí-rè-bìng zhě bí xiān chì. Zhè-xiē yǒu qí zhǔn-què de yī miàn, dàn bù néng zhí cǐ yī duān lùn-dìng.

Lín-zhèng shàng cháng-jiàn de: miàn-bù sè qīng, wéi xiǎo-ér jí-jīng, wéi tán-chuǎn zhòng-zhèng; qīng hēi wéi hán tòng; sè bái wéi qì-xū, wéi wáng-xuè; sè huáng wéi shī-qì, jiān mù huáng wéi huáng-dǎn; sè chì wéi gān-huǒ-shàng-nì, wéi yáng-míng shí-rè, sè chì dú jiàn liǎng quán zhě wéi yīn-xū huǒ-kàng; sè hēi wéi shuǐ-qì, wéi nǚ-láo-dǎn, fù-nǚ yǎn-kuàng sì-zhōu sè hēi zhě wéi dài-xià-bìng.

Vocabulary 10.2

察色	chá-sè	inspect a color
分配	fēn-pèi	associate separately with
部	bù	region
主	zhǔ	rule; indicate

肝热病	gān-rè-bìng	liver heat illness
颊	jiá	lateral cheek
肺热病	fèi-rè-bìng	lung heat illness
心热病	xīn-rè-bìng	heart heat illness
颜	yán	forehead
肾热病	shèn-rè-bìng	kidney heat illness
脾热病	pí-rè-bìng	spleen heat illness
准确	zhǔn-què	real; realistic
执	zhí	cling to
端	duān	end; point; (measure word)
论定	lùn-dìng	definitive statement
急惊	jí-jīng	acute fright
痰喘	tán-chuǎn	phlegm panting
重症	zhòng-zhèng	serious pathocondition
气虚	qì-xū	qi depletion
黄疸	huáng-dǎn	jaundice
肝火上逆	gān-huǒ-shàng-nì	adversely rising liver fire
实热	shí-rè	repletion heat
独	dú	alone; only
火亢	huǒ-kàng	hyperactivity of fire
水气	shuǐ-qì	water qi
女劳疸	nǚ-láo-dǎn	exhaustion resulting from sexual intemperance
妇女	fù-nǚ	woman
四周	sì-zhōu	in all four directions; all around
带下病	dài-xià-bìng	illness below the belt; gynecological illness

Translation 10.2

2. The complexion: To inspect (a patient's) color includes (an examination) of the skin of (his/her) face and of the entire body. (Among the colors) the five types of virid, red, yellow, white, and black are distinguished; each of them is associated, in accordance with the five

phases theory, with one of the five depots. In addition, each of the internal depots is linked to one of the various regions of the face. For example, red is the color of fire; it indicates heat. Hence (Chinese medicine) assumes (the following:) In case of a liver heat illness the left lateral cheek turns red first, in case of a lung heat illness the right lateral cheek turns red first, in case of a heart heat illness the forehead turns red first, in case of a kidney heat illness the cheeks turn red first, and in case of a spleen heat illness the nose turns red first. Although these (assumptions) have their realistic aspects, (a therapist) must not cling to just one (of them as a) definitive statement. (The following situations) are frequently seen in clinical practice: A virid color in the facial region indicates acute fright in infants, and it is (also a sign of) the serious pathocondition of phlegm panting. A virid-black (coloring) indicates cold and pain. A white color indicates qi depletion, and loss of blood. A yellow color indicates (the presence of) dampness qi; if the eyes are yellow too, this indicates jaundice. A red color indicates an adverse rise of liver fire, and (it indicates) repletion heat in the yang brilliance (conduit). If a red color is observed only at the two cheeks, this indicates a yin depletion and a hyperactivity of fire. A black color indicates (the presence of) water qi, and it is (also a sign of) exhaustion resulting from sexual intemperance. If the eye-sockets of women are black all around, this indicates a gynecological illness.

Text 10.3

3. 舌苔：察舌是望诊中重要的一环。舌和苔的定义：舌是舌质，苔是舌质上的一层薄垢，有如地上所长的莓苔，故称舌苔。看舌质是辨别脏气的虚实，看舌苔可以辨别胃气的清浊和外感时邪的性质。总的说来，观察舌质和舌苔的变化，能知疾病的性质及正气和邪气的消长情况。其次，当知舌苔的分部。以五脏来分，舌尖属心，舌根属肾，中心属肺胃，两旁属肝胆。察舌是相当细致的，舌与苔须分看，又须合看。

Transliteration 10.3

3. Shé-tāi: chá-shé shì wàng-zhěn zhōng zhòng-yào de yī huán. Shé hé tāi de dìng-yì: shé shì shé-zhì, tāi shì shé-zhì shàng de yī céng bó gòu, yǒu rú dì shàng suǒ zhǎng de méi-tāi, gù chēng shé-tāi. Kàn shé-zhì shì biàn-bié zàng-qì de xū shí, kàn shé-tāi kě-yǐ biàn-bié wèi-qì de qīng zhuó hé wài-gǎn shí-xié de xìng-zhì. Zǒng-de-shuō-lái, guān-chá shé-zhì hé shé-tāi de biàn-huà, néng zhī jí-bìng de xìng-zhì jí zhèng-qì hé xié-qì de xiāo-zhǎng qíng-kuàng.

Qí-cì, dāng zhī shé-tāi de fēn-bù. Yǐ wǔ-zàng lái fēn, shé-jiān shǔ xīn, shé-gēn shǔ shèn, zhōng-xīn shǔ fèi wèi, liǎng páng shǔ gān dǎn. Chá-shé shì xiāng-dāng xì-zhì de, shé yǔ tāi xū fēn kàn, yòu xū hé kàn.

Vocabulary 10.3

察舌	chá-shé	inspection of the tongue
环	huán	link (in a chain)
苔	tāi	coating
定义	dìng-yì	define
层	céng	layer
薄	bó	thin
垢	gòu	staining
莓苔	méi-tāi	moss coating
脏气	zàng-qì	qi in the depots
时邪	shí-xié	seasonal evil
其次	qí-cì	furthermore; next
分部	fēn-bù	individual regions
舌尖	shé-jiān	tip of the tongue
舌根	shé-gēn	base of the tongue
中心	zhōng-xīn	center
旁	páng	side
合	hé	together

Translation 10.3

3. The tongue-coating: Inspection of the tongue is an important link in the visual examination (of a patient). The definition of tongue and coating (is as follows): tongue is the tongue substance; coating is a layer of thin staining on the tongue substance. (The latter) resembles a moss coating growing on the earth; hence it is named tongue moss. The tongue substance is inspected to distinguish between depletion and repletion of the qi in the depots; by looking at the tongue coating it is possible to distinguish whether the stomach qi is clear or turbid, and (to assess) the nature of a seasonal evil contracted from the outside. Generally speaking, by inspecting the changes of the tongue substance and of the tongue coating it is possible to recognize the nature of an illness, and the circumstances of the waning and growing of proper qi and evil qi.

Furthermore, it is essential to know the individual regions of the tongue coating. If divided in accordance with the five depots, the tip of the tongue belongs to the heart, the base of the tongue belongs to the kidneys, the center belongs to the lung and to the stomach, while the two sides belong to the liver and to the gallbladder. The inspection of the tongue is a fairly meticulous (procedure). It is necessary to look at the tongue and the coating separately, and also to look at them together.

饮食能使舌苔变色，如初进豆浆，牛奶，多见白腻；饮橘子汁多变淡黄；食青果，酱菜等多变灰黑。这种变色，大多浮在舌苔之上，不关舌质，称为"染舌"，于诊断上不足为据。舌上全部无苔，称作光舌，多为阴虚，光如去膜猪腰，为肝肾阴分极伤。舌苔中间缺少一块，称作剥苔。舌光有裂纹，或舌苔燥裂，均为津液损伤。除了观察舌质和舌苔的颜色外，还要辨别老嫩，干润，软硬，战痿，厚薄，松腻，荣枯，胀瘪。

Transliteration 10.4

Yǐn-shí néng shǐ shé-tāi biàn sè, rú chū jìn dòu-jiāng, niú-nǎi duō jiàn bái nì; yǐn jú-zǐ-zhī duō biàn dàn-huáng; shí qīng-guǒ, jiàng-cài děng duō biàn huī-hēi. Zhè-zhǒng biàn sè, dà-duō fú zài shé-tāi zhī shàng, bù guān shé-zhì, chēng-wéi "rǎn-shé," yú zhěn-duàn shàng bù-zú wéi jù.

Shé shàng quán-bù wú tāi, chēng-zuò guāng-shé, duō wéi yīn-xū, guāng rú qù-mó zhū-yāo, wéi gān shèn yīn-fèn jí shāng. Shé-tāi zhōng-jiān quē-shǎo yī kuài, chēng-zuò bō-tāi. Shé-guāng yǒu liè-wén, huò shé-tāi zào-liè, jūn wéi jīn-yè sǔn-shāng.

Chú-le guān-chá shé-zhì hé shé-tāi de yán-sè wài, hái yào biàn-bié lǎo nèn, gān rùn, ruǎn yìng, zhàn wěi, hòu bó, sōng nì, róng kū, zhàng biě.

Vocabulary 10.4

初	chū	just before
豆浆	dòu-jiāng	soy-bean milk
牛奶	niú-nǎi	cow's milk
橘子汁	jú-zǐ-zhī	orange juice
淡黄	dàn-huáng	pale yellow
青果	qīng-guǒ	olives
酱菜	jiàng-cài	food prepared with soy sauce
灰黑	huī-hēi	gray-black
关	guān	affect; concern
染舌	rǎn-shé	stained tongue
据	jù	evidence
光	guāng	shine
光舌	guāng-shé	shiny tongue
去膜	qù-mó	remove the skin
猪腰	zhū-yāo	pig's kidneys
阴分	yīn-fèn	yin section
块	kuài	piece

剥苔	bō-tāi	peeling coating
舌光	shé-guāng	tongue gloss
裂纹	liè-wén	crackles
颜色	yán-sè	color
老	lǎo	aged
嫩	nèn	tender
硬	yìng	hard
战	zhàn	mobile
痿	wěi	stiff
松	sōng	dry; flaky
荣	róng	flourishing
枯	kū	withered
瘪	biě	shrivelled

Translation 10.4

Drink and food can cause the color of the tongue coating to change; for instance, immediately after an intake of soy-bean milk or cow's milk often a white slime appears (on the tongue). Drinking orange juice often changes (the tongue coating) to pale yellow. Eating olives or food prepared with soy sauce often changes (the tongue coating to) gray-black. These kinds of color changes mostly float on top of the tongue coating; they do not affect the tongue substance. (These phenomena) are called "stained tongue"; they do not offer sufficient evidence to arrive at a diagnostic decision.

If there is no coating on the entire tongue, this is called "shiny tongue"; it is often (a sign of) yin depletion. If (the tongue) shines like a pig's kidney after the skin was removed, this indicates a very serious harm in the yin section of liver and kidneys. If a piece is missing in the middle of the tongue coating, this is called "peeling coating." If the tongue gloss shows crackles, or if the tongue coating is cracked because of dryness, all this indicates that the body liquids have been harmed.

In addition to inspecting the tongue substance and the color of the tongue coating, (a therapist) should also distinguish whether it is aged or tender, dry or moist, soft or hard, mobile or stiff, thick or thin, flaky or slimy, flourishing or withered, or swollen or shrivelled.

4. 形态：观察病人的形体姿态动作，对于诊断上也有很大的帮助。如肥人多痰湿，瘦人多内热；一臂不举为痹，半身不遂为中风；膝部屈伸不便，行时偻俯，为筋病；不能久立，行时振掉为骨病；卧时身轻能转侧的为阳病，身重不能转侧的为阴病；常屈一足或蜷曲而卧的多为腹痛症；循衣摸床，撮空理线，为神气散乱。

5. 其它部分：目赤为热，目黄为黄疸，目斜视者多为肝风。鼻塞流涕为感冒，鼻孔干燥，黑如煤熏为阳毒热深，鼻孔煽张为肺风或肺绝。口噤不语为痉，口角歪斜为中风。

Transliteration 10.5

4. Xíng-tài: guān-chá bìng-rén de xíng-tǐ zī-tài dòng-zuò, duì-yú zhěn-duàn shàng yě yǒu hěn dà de bāng-zhù. Rú féi rén duō tán shī, shòu rén duō nèi-rè; yī bì bù jǔ wéi bì, bàn-shēn-bù-suí wéi zhòng-fēng; xī-bù qū shēn bù biàn, xíng shí lǚ fǔ, wéi jīn-bìng; bù néng jiǔ lì, xíng shí zhèn-diào wéi gǔ-bìng; wò shí shēn qīng néng zhuǎn-cè de wéi yáng-bìng, shēn zhòng bù néng zhuǎn-cè de wéi yīn-bìng; cháng qū yī zú huò quán-qū ér wò de duō wéi fù-tòng zhèng; xún-yī mō-chuáng, cuō-kōng lǐ-xiàn, wéi shén-qì sǎn-luàn.

5. Qí-tā bù-fèn: mù-chì wéi rè, mù huáng wéi huáng-dǎn, mù xié-shì zhě duō wéi gān-fēng. Bí-sè liú-tì wéi gǎn-mào, bí-kǒng gān-zào, hēi rú méi-xūn wéi yáng dú-rè shēn, bí-kǒng shān-zhāng wéi fèi-fēng huò fèi-jué. Kǒu-jìn-bù-yǔ wéi jìng, kǒu-jiǎo wāi-xié wéi zhòng-fēng.

Vocabulary 10.5

姿态	zī-tài	posture
动作	dòng-zuò	movement
内热	nèi-rè	inner heat
臂	bì	arm
举	jǔ	lift
痹	bì	paralysis
膝部	xī-bù	knee
偻	lǚ	bent
俯	fǔ	bent

筋病	jīn-bìng	sinew illness
立	lì	stand
振掉	zhèn-diào	sway
骨病	gǔ-bìng	bone illness
蜷曲	quán-qū	bent
循衣	xún-yī	follow the clothes (with the hands)
摸床	mō-chuáng	touch gently the bedding
撮空	cuō-kōng	grasp into the empty (air)
理线	lǐ-xiàn	order threads
神气	shén-qì	spirit qi
散乱	sǎn-luàn	disturbed
斜视	xié-shì	squint
肝风	gān-fēng	liver wind
煤熏	méi-xūn	soot
毒热	dú-rè	poison heat
煽张	shān-zhāng	be widened in excitement
肺风	fèi-fēng	lung wind
肺绝	fèi-jué	lung failure
口噤不语	kǒu-jìn-bù-yǔ	clenched jaw and inability to speak
痉	jìng	spasm
口角	kǒu-jiǎo	corner of the mouth

Translation 10.5

4. The physical shape: Inspecting the posture and movement of the patient's physical body is also of very great help for diagnosis. For instance, obese persons often (carry) phlegm and dampness (in their body); emaciated persons often have internal heat. If one arm cannot be lifted, this is paralysis; hemiplegia is (the result of a) wind stroke. If bending and stretching of the knees is uncomfortable, and if (the patient) is bent forward when walking, these are illnesses of the sinews. If (the patient) cannot stand for long, and if he/she walks unsteadily, that is an

illness of the bones. If the body while lying feels light, and is able to turn sides, it is a yang illness; if the body feels heavy and cannot turn sides, it is a yin illness. If (the patient) frequently crooks one foot or bends himself while lying, that is often a (sign of a) pathocondition of abdominal pain. If (the patient) moves along his/her clothes or touches gently his/her bedding, if he/she grasps into the empty (air) or orders (imaginary) threads, this is (a sign of) a disturbance of his/her spirit qi.

5. Other sections: Red eyes are (indicators of) heat. Yellow eyes indicate jaundice. Squint often indicates liver wind. A congested or running nose indicates a common cold. If the nostrils are desiccated, and if they are black as if sooted, that indicates that poison heat has deeply entered the yang (region). If the nostrils are widened in excitement, that is (a sign of) lung wind or pulmonary failure. Clenched jaw and inability to speak indicates a spasm. If the corners of the mouth are wry, that is (a sign of) wind stroke.

Text 10.6

闻诊分两方面，一方面用听觉来听取病人的语言，呼吸，咳嗽和其它声音的高低，清浊等；另一方面用嗅觉来辨别口气，病气和二便等气味。

1. 声音：语气低微为内伤虚症；细语反复为神思不足；妄言谵语为热盛神昏；高声骂詈，不避亲疏，为癫狂症。呼吸微弱为正虚；气粗为肺胃有热；呼多吸少为痰阻；喉间如拉锯声为痰喘症；吸气困难，似欲断绝，但得引长一息为快者，为肾虚不能纳气；时作叹息，多为情怀不畅。

Transliteration 10.6

Wén-zhěn fèn liǎng fāng-miàn, yī fāng-miàn yòng tīng-jué lái tīng-qǔ bìng-rén de yǔ-yán, hū-xī, ké-sòu hé qí-tā shēng-yīn de gāo-dī, qīng zhuó děng; lìng-yī fāng-miàn yòng xiù-jué lái biàn-bié kǒu-qì, bìng-qì hé èr-biàn děng qì-wèi.

1. Shēng-yīn: yǔ-qì dī wēi wéi nèi-shāng xū-zhèng; xì yǔ fǎn-fù wéi shén-sī bù-zú; wàng-yán zhān-yǔ wéi rè-shèng shén-hūn; gāo shēng mà-lì, bù bì qīn shū, wéi diān-kuáng zhèng.

Hū-xī wēi ruò wéi zhèng xū; qì cū wéi fèi wèi yǒu rè; hū duō xī shǎo wéi tán-zǔ; hóu jiān rú lā-jù shēng wéi tán-chuǎn zhèng; xī qì kùn-nán, sì yù duàn-jué, dàn dé yǐn-cháng yī xī wéi kuài zhě, wéi shèn-xū bù néng nà qì; shí zuò tàn-xī, duō wéi qíng-huái bù chàng.

Vocabulary 10.6

闻诊	wén-zhěn	examination by listening and smelling
听觉	tīng-jué	sense of hearing
听取	tīng-qǔ	listen
高低	gāo-dī	high and low; level
嗅觉	xiù-jué	sense of smelling
口气	kǒu-qì	breath
病气	bìng-qì	qi (odors) emitted by an illness
二便	èr-biàn	stools and urine
气味	qì-wèi	smell
语气	yǔ-qì	intonation
低	dī	deep
语	yǔ	language; speech
妄言	wàng-yán	wild talk
热盛	rè-shèng	extreme heat
声	shēng	sound

骂詈	mà-lì	curse
避	bì	avoid
亲	qīn	relatives
疏	shū	distant
癫狂	diān-kuáng	mania and/or depression
粗	cū	rough
痰阻	tán-zǔ	phlegm obstruction
拉锯	lā-jù	bow saw
困难	kùn-nán	difficulty
断绝	duàn-jué	stop; break off
引长	yǐn-cháng	protract
息	xī	breathing
快	kuài	happy; comfortable
纳	nà	take in
时	shí	from time to time
叹息	tàn-xī	sigh
情怀	qíng-huái	emotion
畅	chàng	unimpeded; unconstrained

Translation 10.6

The examination by listening and smelling is divided into two aspects. On the one side the sense of hearing is used to listen to the level, to the clarity and so on of the patient's language, breathing, coughing, and other sounds. On the other side, the sense of smelling is used to differentiate among the smells of (the patient's) breath, of the qi (odors emitted by his/her) illness, and of stools and urine.

1. The sounds: An intonation that is deep and feeble is a pathocondition of internal harm and depletion. A recurring thin speech is (a sign of) a weakened mind. Wild talk and incoherent language indicate extreme heat and mental disturbance. Cursing with a high voice, regardless of whether relatives or more distant (persons) are concerned, is a pathocondition of mania and/or depression.

When the breathing is feeble and weak, this is a (sign of) depletion of the proper (qi). If the breath is rough, this indicates that the lung and the stomach have heat. If exhalation is increased in comparison with inhalation, this indicates phlegm stagnation. If there is a sound in the throat resembling (the movement of) a bow saw, this is a pathocondition of phlegm panting. If (the patient) has difficulty inhaling air, if it seems as if (his/her breath) were to stop, and if he/she feels comfortable only when he/she protracts each single breathing, then these are (signs of) a kidney depletion, (the latter) being unable to take in qi. If (the patient) sighs from time to time, this is often (a sign of) constrained emotions.

2.气味：口内出气秽臭的为胃有湿热；嗳气带酸腐气的为胃有宿食；痰有腥秽气的为肺热；臭甚而咯出脓样者为肺痈。大便酸臭溏薄为肠有积热食滞；小便腥臭浑浊为膀胱湿热；矢气奇臭，多为消化不良。病气，就是病人所特有的一种酸臭的秽气，常见于时病热症及瘟疫病。体弱者闻之极易感染。如温病得汗，身热不解，先有汗酸臭；当发疹发斑时期，其气更重。瘟疫病则一开始即有病气触鼻。

Transliteration 10.7

2. Qì-wèi: kǒu-nèi chū qì huì chòu de wéi wèi yǒu shī-rè; ǎi-qì dài suān fǔ qì de wéi wèi yǒu sù-shí; tán yǒu xīng huì qì de wéi fèi-rè; chòu shèn ér kǎ-chū nóng yàng zhě wéi fèi-yōng.

Dà-biàn suān chòu táng-bó wéi cháng yǒu jī-rè shí-zhì; xiǎo-biàn xīng-chòu hún-zhuó wéi páng-guāng shī-rè; shǐ-qì qí chòu, duō wéi xiāo-huà bù-liáng.

Bìng-qì, jiù-shì bìng-rén suǒ tè-yǒu de yī zhǒng suān chòu de huì qì, cháng jiàn yú shí-bìng rè-zhèng jí wēn-yì-bìng. Tǐ ruò zhě wén zhī jí yì gǎn-rǎn. Rú wēn-bìng dé hàn, shēn-rè bù jiě, xiān yǒu hàn suān chòu; dāng fā-zhěn fā-bān shí-qī, qí qì gèng zhòng. Wēn-yì-bìng zé yī kāi-shǐ jí yǒu bìng-qì chù bí.

Vocabulary 10.7

口内	kǒu-nèi	interior of the mouth
出	chū	leave
臭	chòu	fetid
嗳气	ǎi-qì	belching
带	dài	carry along
腐	fǔ	putrid
宿食	sù-shí	undigested food
腥	xīng	rotten smell
咯出	kǎ-chū	cough up
样	yàng	type
肺痈	fèi-yōng	lung abscess
积热	jī-rè	heat accumulation
食滞	shí-zhì	food blockage
腥臭	xīng-chòu	rotten-fetid
浑浊	hún-zhuó	turbid
矢气	shǐ-qì	flatulence
奇	qí	extraordinarily

时病	shí-bìng	seasonal illness
瘟疫病	wēn-yì-bìng	infectious epidemic illness
解	jiě	solve; end
开始	kāi-shǐ	begin
触	chù	strike; rise to

Translation 10.7

2. Smells: If the breath leaving the mouth has an impure fetid (smell), that is (a sign of) dampness heat in the stomach. Belching of sour putrid air indicates that the stomach holds undigested food. Phlegm emitting rotten fetid air indicates lung heat. Very fetid (phlegm) that is coughed up and resembles pus indicates a pulmonary abscess.

Sour fetid and semiliquid stool is (a sign of) heat accumulations and food blockages in the intestines. Rotten-fetid and turbid urine indicates dampness heat in the bladder. Flatulence smelling extraordinarily fetid is often a (sign of) poor digestion.

The (above-mentioned) qi (odors emitted by an) illness are a kind of sour fetid, impure air that is characteristic of patients. It appears often in conjunction with heat pathoconditions of seasonal illnesses, and also in conjunction with infectious epidemic diseases. If physically weakened (persons) inhale these (odors), they are most easily infected (themselves). For instance, if in case of an epidemic febrile disease (the patient) must sweat, and if his/her fever does not end, (the patient's) sweat will smell sour fetid at first. Once (the patient) develops papules or macules, these qi (odors) will be even stronger. (That is,) as soon as an infectious epidemic disease begins (to develop), qi (odors emitted by this) illness will strike the nose.

Text 10.8

诊病必须了解病人的生活习惯，精神状态以及发病，转变的情况，必要时还得了解其家族史及个人的已往病史。一般在临症上都以发病过程和自觉症状为主要的问诊内容，问诊时有一定的程序，张景岳曾作十问歌："一问寒热二问汗，三问头身四问便，五问饮食六问胸，七聋八渴俱当辨，九因脉色察阴阳，十从气味章神见"。十问里包括了外感和内伤的辨别。

Transliteration 10.8

Zhěn bìng bì-xū liǎo-jiě bìng-rén de shēng-huó xí-guàn, jīng-shén-zhuàng-tài yǐ-jí fā-bìng, zhuǎn-biàn de qíng-kuàng, bì-yào shí hái dé liǎo-jiě qí jiā-zú shǐ jí gè-rén de yǐ-wǎng bìng shǐ. Yī-bān zài lín-zhèng shàng dōu yǐ fā-bìng guò-chéng hé zì-jué zhèng-zhuàng wéi zhǔ-yào de wèn-zhěn nèi-róng, wèn-zhěn shí yǒu yī-dìng de chéng-xù, zhāng jǐng-yuè zēng zuò shí-wèn-gē: "Yī wèn hán rè èr wèn hàn, sān wèn tóu shēn sì wèn biàn, wǔ wèn yǐn-shí liù wèn xiōng, qī lóng bā kě jù dāng biàn, jiǔ yīn mài sè chá yīn yáng, shí cóng qì wèi zhāng shén-jiàn. "Shí-wèn lǐ bāo-kuò le wài-gǎn hé nèi-shāng de biàn-bié.

Vocabulary 10.8

了解	liǎo-jiě	understand; find out
习惯	xí-guàn	habits and customs
精神状态	jīng-shén-zhuàng-tài	mental state
转变	zhuǎn-biàn	transformation
家族	jiā-zú	family
史	shǐ	history
个人	gè-rén	each person
已往	yǐ-wǎng	earlier; in the past
觉	jué	perceive; feel
自觉	zì-jué	subjective
问	wèn	ask
问诊	wèn-zhěn	examination by way of asking
张景岳	zhāng jǐng-yuè	(author's name:) Zhang Jingyue
十	shí	ten
十问	shí-wèn	the ten (diagnostic) questions
十问歌	shí-wèn-gē	the Poem of the Ten (diagnostic) Questions
七	qī	seven
聋	lóng	dumb
八	bā	eight

察	chá	examine; investigate
章	zhāng	display
神见	shén-jiàn	perfect understanding

Translation 10.8

To diagnose an illness, it is necessary to be familiar with the habits and customs in the patient's life, with his/her mental state, and with the circumstances of the onset and (later) transformations of the illness. Where necessary, the history of his/her family and of previous illness histories of each (member of the family) should be known too. In general, the most important issues in clinical reality to be discussed, in an examination, by way of asking (the patient) include the process of the emergence of the illness, and the subjective pathoconditions (felt by the patient him/herself). During an examination by way of asking (the patient), a firm sequence (of questions) exists. Formerly, Zhang Jingyue[1] formulated the Poem of the Ten Questions: "First, inquire about cold and heat, then inquire about sweat. Third, inquire about head and body; fourth, inquire about the excrements. Fifth, inquire about eating and drinking; sixth, inquire about the chest. Seventh, hearing and, eighth, thirst must all be distinguished; ninth, inspect the yin and yang on the basis of pulse and complexion, and, tenth, take the smells to display your perfect understanding (of the patient's illness)." These ten questions include (methods for) distinguishing exogenous affections and internal harm.

Note

1 Zhang Jiebin 张介宾 (1563-1640), style name Jingyue, was a famous physician and author of the Ming dynasty.

Text 11.1

切诊以按脉为主，并包括其他触诊在内。

1. 切脉：切脉采取两手寸口即掌后桡骨动脉的部位，用食指，中指和无名指轻按，重按，或单按，总按，以寻求脉象。每手分三部，以掌后高骨作标志，定名为"关"，关之前名"寸"，关之后名"尺"，两手寸关尺共六部，称为左寸，左关，左尺，右寸，右关，右尺。这六部分都是候测内脏之气的。左寸候心和心包络，左关候肝和胆，左尺候肾和膀胱，小肠；右寸候肺，右关候脾和胃，右尺候肾和命门，大肠。

Transliteration 11.1

Qiè-zhěn yǐ àn mài wéi zhǔ, bìng bāo-kuò qí-tā chù-zhěn zài nèi.

1. Qiè-mài: qiè-mài cǎi-qǔ liǎng shǒu cùn-kǒu jí zhǎng hòu náo-gǔ dòng-mài de bù-wèi, yòng shí-zhǐ, zhōng-zhǐ hé wú-míng-zhǐ qīng-àn, zhòng-àn, huò dān-àn, zǒng-àn, yǐ xún-qiú mài-xiàng. Měi shǒu fēn sān-bù, yǐ zhǎng hòu gāo-gǔ zuò biāo-zhì, dìng-míng wéi "guān," guān zhī qián míng "cùn," guān zhī hòu míng "chǐ," liǎng shǒu cùn guān chǐ gòng liù bù, chēng-wéi zuǒ-cùn, zuǒ-guān, zuǒ-chǐ, yòu-cùn, yòu-guān, yòu-chǐ. Zhè liù bù-fen dōu-shì hòu-cè nèi-zàng zhī qì de. Zuǒ-cùn hòu xīn hé xīn-bāo-luò, zuǒ-guān hòu gān hé dǎn, zuǒ-chǐ hòu shèn hé páng-guāng, xiǎo-cháng; yòu-cùn hòu fèi, yòu-guān hòu pí hé wèi, yòu-chǐ hòu shèn hé mìng-mén, dà-cháng.

Vocabulary 11.1

切诊	qiè-zhěn	palpation
按	àn	press; feel (the pulse)
其他	qí-tā	other
触诊	chù-zhěn	examination through touching (the patient)
切脉	qiè-mài	feel the pulse
采取	cǎi-qǔ	select
寸口	cùn-kǒu	inch opening

掌	zhǎng	palm
桡骨	náo-gǔ	radius
动脉	dòng-mài	pulsating vessel
指	zhǐ	finger
食指	shí-zhǐ	index finger
中指	zhōng-zhǐ	middle finger
无名指	wú-míng-zhǐ	ring finger
轻按	qīng-àn	press lightly
重按	zhòng-àn	press heavily
单按	dān-àn	feel with one (finger)
总按	zǒng-àn	feel (with all three fingers) together
寻求	xún-qiú	investigate
三部	sān-bù	the three sections (at the wrists where the pulse can be felt)
高骨	gāo-gǔ	elevated bone
标志	biāo-zhì	characteristic; reference point
作	zuò	serve as
定名	dìng-míng	name
关	guān	pass gate
寸	cùn	inch
尺	chǐ	foot
共	gòng	together
左寸	zuǒ-cùn	left inch
左关	zuǒ-guān	left gate
左尺	zuǒ-chǐ	left foot
右寸	yòu-cùn	right inch
右关	yòu-guān	right gate
右尺	yòu-chǐ	right foot
候	hòu	examine
候测	hòu-cè	assess

Translation 11.1

Palpation consists mainly of feeling the pulse, but includes other examinations by means of touching as well.

1. Pulse feeling: To feel the pulse at both hands the inch opening, i.e., the location of the pulsating vessel at the radius behind the palm, is selected to exert light or heavy pressure with the index finger, the middle finger, and the ring finger, either with one (finger alone) or with all (fingers together), to investigate the appearance of the pulse. At each hand three sections are distinguished. The elevated bone behind the palm is the reference point; it is named "pass gate[1]". (The section) in front of the gate is named "inch"; (the section) behind the pass gate is called "foot[2]." Inch, pass gate, and foot (sections) of both hands together constitute six sections; they are called left inch, left pass gate, left foot, right inch, right pass gate, and right foot. All these six sections (serve) to assess the qi of the inner depots. At the left inch the heart and the heart-enclosing network are investigated; at the left pass gate the liver and the gallbladder are investigated; at the left foot the kidneys and the bladder as well as the small intestine are investigated. At the right inch the lung is investigated; at the right pass gate the spleen and the stomach are investigated; and at the right foot the kidneys and the gate of life as well as the large intestine are investigated.

Notes

1 At the level of the styloid processus is an imaginative line called "pass gate," possibly because this is the borderline between the yang section and the yin section.

2 "Inch" and "foot" are measures of length. These terms indicate the tenfold length of the distances suitable for feeling the pulse, while the middle finger palpates the "pass gate." One (= odd number = yang) tenth of an inch corresponds to the yang section reaching from the pass gate upwards (in the direction of the palm); ten (= even number = yin) tenths of an inch (= 1 foot) corresponds to the yin section reaching from the pass gate downwards, into the direction of the elbow.

Text 11.2

一般的说，脉象分二十八种，它的名称是：浮，沉，迟，数，滑，涩，虚，实，长，短，洪，微，紧，缓，芤，弦，革，牢，濡，弱，细，散，伏，动，促，结，代，疾。这些脉象，大多是相对的，如以浮和沉分表里，迟和数分寒热，涩和滑分虚实，其它均从这六脉化出。例如：浮而极有力，如按鼓皮为革；浮而极无力，如绵在水为濡。沉而按之着骨始得为伏；沉而坚实为牢；沉而无力，细按乃得为弱。浮中沉均有力，应指愊愊然为实；浮中沉均无力，应指豁豁然为虚；浮取大，按之中空，如慈葱为芤。

Transliteration 11.2

Yī-bān-de-shuō, mài-xiàng fēn èr-shí-bā zhǒng, tā-de míng-chēng shì: fú, chén, chí, shuò, huá, sè, xū, shí, cháng, duǎn, hóng, wēi, jǐn, huǎn, kōu, xián, gé, láo, rú, ruò, xì, sàn, fú, dòng, cù, jié, dài, jí. Zhè-xiē mài-xiàng, dà-duō shì xiāng-duì de, rú yǐ fú hé chén fēn biǎo lǐ, chí hé shuò fēn hán rè, sè hé huá fēn xū shí, qí-tā jūn cóng zhè liù mài huà-chū. Lì-rú: fú ér jí yǒu-lì, rú àn gǔ-pí wéi gé; fú ér jí wú-lì, rú mián zài shuǐ wéi rú. Chén ér àn zhī zháo gǔ shǐ dé wéi fú; chén ér jiān shí wéi láo; chén ér wú-lì, xì àn nǎi dé wéi ruò. Fú zhōng chén jūn yǒu-lì, yīng zhǐ bí-bì-rán wéi shí; fú zhōng chén jūn wú-lì, yīng zhǐ huò-huò-rán wéi xū; fú qǔ dà, àn zhī zhōng kōng, rú cí-cōng wéi kōu.

Vocabulary 11.2

二十八	èr-shí-bā	twenty eight
虚	xū	depleted (pulse condition)
实	shí	replete (pulse condition)
长	cháng	extended (pulse condition)
芤	kōu	(pulse condition resembling a) scallion stalk: hard outside, hollow inside
革	gé	tympanic (pulse condition)
牢	láo	tethered (pulse condition)
濡	rú	soft (pulse condition)

促	cù	hasty (pulse condition)
代	dài	intermittent (pulse condition)
疾	jí	hurried (pulse condition)
相对	xiāng-duì	be mutually opposite
化出	huà-chū	derive by modification
有力	yǒu-lì	have strength; strong
鼓皮	gǔ-pí	drum skin
绵	mián	silk floss
着	zháo	reach; get to; press against
愊愊然	bī-bī-rán	pressing; forceful
应	yīng	respond (to the pressure of a finger)
始	shǐ	begin
乃	nǎi	hence (often untranslatable)
然	rán	like; as if
豁豁然	huò-huò-rán	fragile; breakable
取	qǔ	get (something as a result of an investigation); notice
空	kōng	empty
慈葱	cí-cōng	tender spring onion

Translation 11.2

Generally speaking, 28 types of pulse condition are distinguished. Their names are: at the surface, deep, retarded, accelerated, soft, rough, depleted, replete, extended, short, vast, feeble, tense, relaxed, scallion stalk, string-like, tympanic, tethered, soft, weak, fine, dispersed, hidden, tremulous, hasty, knotty, intermittent, and hurried. Most of these pulse appearances are mutually opposed. For example, by means of (the pulses appearing) "at the surface" and "deep," (therapists) distinguish between (illnesses located in) the outside and in the inside (of the body). By means of (pulses appearing) "retarded" and "accelerated," cold and heat are distinguished; and by means of (pulses appearing) "rough" and "soft," depletion and repletion are distinguished. All the other (pulse appearances) are modifications of these six pulses. For instance, if (a pulse) is at the surface and very strong, and if it feels like touching a drum skin, this is a tympanic (pulse). If (a pulse) is at the surface and has no strength at all, resembling silk floss in water, this is a soft (pulse). If (a pulse) is deep, and if (the therapist) has to press down to the bone to get a hold of it, this is a hidden (pulse). If (a pulse) is deep and if it is solid and replete, this is a tethered (pulse). If it is deep and has no strength, and if it is felt by exerting mild pressure, this is a weak (pulse). If it has strength at the surface, in the center, and deep, and responds to the finger with force, this is a replete (pulse). If it has no strength at the surface, in the center, and deep, and if it responds to the finger as if breaking, this is a depleted (pulse). If a strong (pulse) is felt at the surface, and if it is empty in the center under pressure, resembling a tender spring onion, this is a scallion-stalk (pulse).

迟而细短，往来涩滞为涩；一息四至，往来和匀为缓；缓而时止为结；数而在关，无头无尾为动；数而时一止为促；每一息七至八至为疾；迟数不定，止有常数为代；至数不齐，按之浮乱为散。滑而如按琴弦为弦；来往有力如转索为紧；不小不大，如循长竿为长；来盛去衰，来大去长为洪；涩而极细软，按之欲绝为微；如微而细为细；如豆形应指即回为短。因此，浮沉，迟数，涩滑是二十八脉的纲领，学习切脉应当先从这六个纲领入手，比较容易体会和理解。

Transliteration 11.3

Chí ér xì duǎn, wǎng-lái sè zhì wéi sè; yī xī sì zhì, wǎng-lái hé yún wéi huǎn; huǎn ér shí zhǐ wéi jié; shuò ér zài guān, wú tóu wú wěi wéi dòng; shuò ér shí yī zhǐ wéi cù; měi yī xī qī zhì bā zhì wéi jí; chí shuò bù-dìng, zhǐ yǒu cháng-shù wéi dài; zhì-shù bù qí, àn zhī fú luàn wéi sàn. Huá ér rú àn qín-xián wéi xián; lái-wǎng yǒu-lì rú zhuǎn-suǒ wéi jǐn; bù xiǎo bù dà, rú xún cháng gān wéi cháng; lái shèng qù shuāi, lái dà qù cháng wéi hóng; sè ér jí xì ruǎn, àn zhī yù jué wéi wēi; rú wēi ér xì wéi xì; rú dòu xíng yīng zhǐ jí huí wéi duǎn. Yīn-cǐ, fú chén, chí shuò, sè huá shì èr-shí-bā mài de gāng-lǐng, xué-xí qiè-mài yīng-dāng xiān cóng zhè liù gè gāng-lǐng rù-shǒu, bǐ-jiào róng-yì tǐ-huì hé lǐ-jiě.

Vocabulary 11.3

和	hé	balanced
匀	yún	even
止	zhǐ	stop
尾	wěi	tail
常数	cháng-shù	constant; regularly
齐	qí	regular
琴弦	qín-xián	lute string
来往	lái-wǎng	come and go
转索	zhuǎn-suǒ	twisted rope
小	xiǎo	small
竿	gān	cane
衰	shuāi	weak

绝	jué	break off
豆	dòu	bean
回	huí	return
从 ... 入手	cóng ... rù-shǒu	start from ...

Translation 11.3

If (the pulse) is retarded, as well as fine and short, and if it comes and goes rough and haltingly, this is a rough (pulse). If during one breathing (period) four (pulse beats) arrive, and if these (pulse beats) come and go balanced and evenly, this is a relaxed (pulse). If it is relaxed and stops at times, this is a knotted (pulse). If it is accelerated and can be felt at the gate, and if it has no head and no tail, then it is tremulous. If it is accelerated and stops at times, it is hasty. If it comes seven or eight times during one breathing (period), it is hurried. If it is retarded or accelerated for undeterminable (periods), and if it stops regularly, this is an intermittent (pulse). If the arrival frequency is irregular, and if pressing it (shows it to be) at the surface and disorderly, this is a dispersed (pulse). If it is soft and feels like pressing a lute string, this is a string(-like pulse). If it comes and goes with force, resembling a twisted rope, this is a tense (pulse). If it is neither small nor large, and if it feels as if (the fingers) followed a long cane, this is an extended (pulse). If it comes abounding and leaves weakened, if it comes large and leaves extended, this is a vast (pulse). If it is rough and extremely fine as well as soft, and if under pressure it (seems as if it) were about to be interrupted, this is a feeble (pulse). If it is like a feeble (pulse) and fine, this is a fine (pulse). If it resembles the shape of a bean, and if it responds to the finger by immediate retreat, this is a short (pulse). Hence "at the surface" and "deep," "retarded" and "accelerated," as well as "rough" and "soft" are the ordering principles of the 28 pulses. For the study of pulse feeling, it is appropriate to begin with these six ordering principles; they are relatively easy to learn and to understand.

Text 11.4

诸脉各有形象，各有主症，因多错综出现，必须进一步探求，才能应用于临症。如：浮紧为伤寒，浮缓为中风，浮虚为伤暑，浮芤为失血，浮数为风热。沉细为虚寒，沉数为内热，沉紧为冷痛，沉弦为伏饮，沉迟为痼冷。浮迟为表寒，沉迟为里寒，迟涩为血少，迟缓为寒湿。滑数为实热，弦滑为肝火，细滑为阴虚内热，浮滑为风痰，沉滑为宿食，滑大为胃热。这都是显示邪正的盛衰，病邪的性质和发病的部位，故必须与症候密切结合，观察其是否脉症符合为要。

Transliteration 11.4

Zhū mài gè yǒu xíng-xiàng, gè yǒu zhǔ-zhèng, yīn duō cuò-zōng chū-xiàn, bì-xū jìn-yī-bù tàn-qiú, cái néng yìng-yòng yú lín-zhèng. Rú: fú jǐn wéi shāng-hán, fú huǎn wéi zhòng-fēng, fú xū wéi shāng-shǔ, fú kōu wéi shī-xuè, fú shuò wéi fēng-rè. Chén xì wéi xū-hán, chén shuò wéi nèi-rè, chén jǐn wéi lěng-tòng, chén xián wéi fú-yǐn, chén chí wéi gù-lěng. Fú chí wéi biǎo-hán, chén chí wéi lǐ-hán, chí sè wéi xuè-shǎo, chí huǎn wéi hán-shī. Huá shuò wéi shí-rè, xián huá wéi gān-huǒ, xì huá wéi yīn-xū nèi-rè, fú huá wéi fēng-tán, chén huá wéi sù-shí, huá dà wéi wèi-rè. Zhè dōu-shì xiǎn-shì xié zhèng de shèng-shuāi, bìng-xié de xìng-zhì hé fā-bìng de bù-wèi, gù bì-xū yǔ zhèng-hòu mì-qiè jié-hé, guān-chá qí shì-fǒu mài zhèng fú-hé wéi yào.

Vocabulary 11.4

诸	zhū	all
形象	xíng-xiàng	physical appearance
探求	tàn-qiú	search; investigate
伤暑	shāng-shǔ	harm from summerheat
虚寒	xū-hán	depletion cold
冷痛	lěng-tòng	cold pain
伏饮	fú-yǐn	hidden drinks
痼冷	gù-lěng	obstinate frigidity
表寒	biǎo-hán	outside cold
里寒	lǐ-hán	internal cold
血少	xuè-shǎo	diminished blood
寒湿	hán-shī	cold damp
胃热	wèi-rè	stomach heat
显示	xiǎn-shì	show; be a sign of

是否	shì-fǒu ...	whether; whether ... or not
符合	fú-hé	be in keeping with; coincide

Translation 11.4

All pulses have (their specific) physical appearance, and they all have their main pathoconditions (for which they stand). Since (different pulses) often appear mixed up, some additional investigations must be conducted before (the results of pulse feeling) can be applied in clinical practice. For example, (a pulse that is) at the surface and tense indicates harm caused by cold; (a pulse that is) at the surface and relaxed indicates (the patient was) struck by wind. (One that is) at the surface and depleted indicates harm caused by summerheat; (one that is) at the surface and (resembles a) scallion stalk indicates a loss of blood. (One that is) at the surface and accelerated indicates wind-heat. (One that is) deep and fine indicates depletion-cold; (one that is) deep and accelerated indicates internal heat. (One that is) deep and tense indicates cold pain; (one that is) deep and string(-like) indicates deep-lying drink.[1] (One that is) deep and retarded indicates obstinate frigidity. (One that is) at the surface and retarded indicates inside cold. (One that is) retarded and rough indicates diminished blood; (one that is) retarded and relaxed indicates cold damp. (One that is) soft and accelerated indicates repletion heat; (one that is) string(-like) and soft indicates liver fire. (One that is) fine and smooth indicates yin depletion and internal heat. (One that is) at the surface and smooth indicates wind phlegm; (one that is) deep and smooth indicates undigested food. (One that is) smooth and large indicates stomach heat. All these (pulses) indicate an abundance or weakness of evil and proper (qi), the nature of the pathogenic evil, and the location where the illness develops. Hence they are to be closely associated with the pathoconditions and symptoms, and it is essential to investigate whether the pulses are in keeping with the pathoconditions or not.

Note

1 The notion of "deep-lying drink" in the body serves to interpret a syndrom including such symptoms as repeated back pain; fullness; pressure in the realm of chest and diaphragm, coughing, vomiting, fever, and an aversion to cold.

辨别二十八脉不是简单的事，必须通过临症慢慢体会。兹录前人二十八脉总括以便记诵：" 浮行皮肤，沉行肉骨。浮沉既谙，迟数当觉，三至为迟，六至为数。浮沉迟数，各有虚实，无力为虚，有力为实。迟数既明，部位须识，濡浮无力，弱沉无力，沉极为牢，浮极为革，三部皆小，微脉可考，三部皆大，散脉可会，其名曰伏，不见于浮，惟中无力，其名曰芤。部位既明，至数宜晰，四至为缓，七至为疾，数止曰促，缓止曰结。至数既识，形状当别，紧粗而弹，弦细而直，长则迢迢，短则缩缩，谓之洪者，来盛去衰，谓之动者，动摇不移，谓之滑者，流利往来，谓之涩者，进退艰哉，谓之细者，状如丝然，谓之代者，如数止焉。"

Transliteration 11.5

Biàn-bié èr-shí-bā mài bù shì jiǎn-dān de shì, bì-xū tōng-guò lín-zhèng màn-màn tǐ-huì. Zī lù qián-rén èr-shí-bā mài zǒng-kuò yǐ-biàn jì-sòng: "fú xíng pí-fū, chén xíng ròu gǔ. Fú chén jì ān, chí shuò dāng jué, sān zhì wéi chí, liù zhì wéi shuò. Fú chén chí shuò, gè yǒu xū shí, wú-lì wéi xū, yǒu-lì wéi shí. Chí shuò jì míng, bù-wèi xū shí, rú fú wú-lì, ruò chén wú-lì, chén-jí wéi láo, fú-jí wéi gé, sān-bù jiē xiǎo, wēi mài kě-kǎo, sān-bù jiē dà, sàn mài kě-huì, qí míng yuē fú, bù jiàn yú fú, wéi zhōng wú-lì, qí míng yuē kōu. Bù-wèi jì míng, zhì-shù yí xī, sì zhì wéi huǎn, qī zhì wéi jí, shuò zhǐ yuē cù, huǎn zhǐ yuē jié. Zhì-shù jì shí, xíng-zhuàng dāng bié, jǐn cū ér dàn, xián xì ér zhí, cháng zé tiáo-tiáo, duǎn zé suō-suō, wèi zhī hóng zhě, lái shèng qù shuāi, wèi zhī dòng zhě, dòng yáo bù yí, wèi zhī huá zhě, liú-lì wǎng-lái, wèi zhī sè zhě, jìn-tuì jiān zāi, wèi zhī xì zhě, zhuàng rú sī rán, wèi zhī dài zhě, rú shuò zhǐ yān."

Vocabulary 11.5

事	shì	affair
慢慢	màn-màn	slow
录	lù	record
总括	zǒng-kuò	survey
便	biàn	easy; facilitate
记诵	jì-sòng	learn by heart
谙	ān	be familiar with something
明	míng	clear
沉极	chén-jí	extremely deep (pulse condition)
浮极	fú-jí	extremely superficial (pulse condition)
可考	kě-kǎo	certainly
可会	kě-huì	definitely
晰	xī	clear
形状	xíng-zhuàng	shape
别	bié	distinguish
弹	dàn	round
迢迢	tiáo-tiáo	stretched; distant
缩缩	suō-suō	shrunken
谓	wèi	name; call
摇	yáo	tremble
流利	liú-lì	flow
进退	jìn-tuì	advance and retreat; come and go
艰	jiān	difficult
哉	zāi	(particle emphasizing the preceding statement)
丝	sī	silk
焉	yān	(final particle)

Translation 11.5

To distinguish the 28 pulses is not an easy affair; it is necessary to reach a slow understanding through clinical practice. (Hence I) record here a survey of the 28 pulses (compiled) by people in former times to facilitate learning them by heart: "At the surface it passes through the skin; deeply it passes through the flesh and the bones. Once it is known whether it is at the surface or deep, (the therapist) must recognize whether it is retarded or accelerated. If it arrives three (times during one breathing period), it is retarded; if it arrives six (times), it is accelerated. (Pulses that are) at the surface and deep, retarded and accelerated may all be depleted or replete. If they have no strength, they are depleted; if they have strength, they are replete. Once it is clear whether (a pulse) is retarded or accelerated, its location (must be comprehended). A soft (pulse) is at the surface and has no strength; a weak (pulse) is deep and has no strength. When it is extremely deep, it is tethered; when it is at the extreme surface, it is tympanic. A small (pulse) in all three sections is certainly a feeble pulse; a large (pulse) in all three sections is definitely a dispersed pulse. When it is called hidden, it does not appear at the surface; if it is only in the middle and has no strength, (then) it is called scallion-stalk. Once the location is clear, the frequency of the arrivals is to be found out. If it arrives four (times per breathing period), it is relaxed; if it arrives seven (times), it is hurried. If it is accelerated and stops (in between), this is called hasty; if it is relaxed and stops (in between), this is called knotted. Once the frequency of the arrivals is known, the appearance (of the pulses) is to be distinguished. A tense (pulse) is rough and round; a string(-like pulse) is fine and straight. An extended (pulse) is stretched long; a short (pulse) is shrunken. Those (pulses) that are called vast, they come abounding and leave weakened; those that are called tremulous, vacillate without moving away. Those that are called smooth, come and go in free flow; those that are called rough, arrive and retreat under difficulties. Those that are called fine, their shape resembles silk threads; those that are called intermittent resemble those that are accelerated, and stop (in between)."

Text 11.6

二十八脉之外，尚有七怪脉：一曰雀啄，连连凑指，顿有顿无，如雀啄食之状；二曰屋漏，如残霤之下，良久一滴，溅起无力；三曰弹石，来坚而促，来迟去速，如指弹石；四曰解索，脉来动数，随即散乱无序；五曰鱼翔，脉来头定而尾摇，浮浮泛泛；六曰虾游，脉在皮肤，如虾游水面，杳然不见，须臾复来；七曰釜沸，有出无入，如汤涌沸。这些脉象均为心脏极度衰竭，表示生机已绝，多属死候。

Transliteration 11.6

Èr-shí-bā mài zhī wài, shàng yǒu qī-guài-mài: yī yuē què-zhuó, lián-lián còu zhǐ, dùn yǒu dùn wú, rú què-zhuó shí zhī zhuàng; èr yuē wū-lòu, rú cán-liú zhī xià, liáng-jiǔ yī dī, jiàn-qǐ wú-lì: sān yuē tán-shí, lái jiān ér cù, lái chí qù sù, rú zhǐ tán-shí; sì yuē jiě-suǒ, mài lái dòng shuò, suí-jí sǎn-luàn wú xù; wǔ yuē yú-xiáng, mài lái tóu dìng ér wěi yáo, fú-fú-fàn-fàn; liù yuē xiā-yóu, mài zài pí-fū, rú xiā-yóu shuǐ-miàn, yǎo rán bù jiàn, xū-yú fù-lái; qī yuē fǔ-fèi, yǒu chū wú rù, rú tāng yǒng fèi. Zhè-xiē mài-xiàng jūn wéi xīn-zàng jí-dù shuāi-jié, biǎo-shì shēng-jī yǐ jué, duō shǔ sǐ hòu.

Vocabulary 11.6

怪	guài	uncommon
七怪脉	qī-guài-mài	the seven uncommon pulses
雀啄	què-zhuó	pecking bird (pulse condition)
连	lián	tie; connect
连连	lián-lián	again and again; in rapid succession
凑	còu	hit
顿	dùn	suddenly
状	zhuàng	appearance
屋漏	wū-lòu	leaking house (pulse condition)
残霤	cán-liù	cracked gutter
良久	liáng-jiǔ	long time
滴	dī	drop
溅起	jiàn-qǐ	splash
弹石	tán-shí	flicking a stone (pulse condition)
速	sù	fast
解索	jiě-suǒ	untying a rope (pulse condition)
随即	suí-jí	soon afterwards
序	xù	order
鱼翔	yú-xiáng	waving fish (pulse condition)

定	dìng	fix
浮浮泛泛	fú-fú-fàn-fàn	float or bob at the surface; superficial and volatile (intensification of meaning through doubling)
虾游	xiā-yóu	swimming shrimp (pulse condition)
水面	shuǐ-miàn	water surface
杳	yǎo	vanish without traces
须臾	xū-yú	moment
复来	fù-lái	return
釜沸	fǔ-fèi	seething cauldron (pulse condition)
沸	fèi	boil; seethe
涌	yǒng	gush forth; well up
极度	jí-dù	extreme
衰竭	shuāi-jié	weakness
表示	biǎo-shì	indicate; be a sign of
生机	shēng-jī	life processes
候	hòu	sign

Translation 11.6

In addition to the 28 pulses, there are the seven uncommon pulses: The first is called "pecking bird." It hits the finger in rapid succession; suddenly it is present, and suddenly it is gone. Its appearance resembles a bird pecking food. The second is called "leaking house." It resembles (water dripping from) underneath a cracked gutter. It takes a long time for a single drop (to form), and it splashes up without strength. The third is called "flicking a stone." It comes hard and hasty; it comes retarded and leaves fast, as if a stone were flicked with a finger. The fourth is called "untying a rope." The pulse comes tremulous and accelerated, and soon afterwards it is dispersed and confused and lacks any order. The fifth is called "waving fish." The pulse comes with the head fixed and with the tail wiggling. It floats at the surface. The sixth is called "swimming shrimp." This pulse is in the skin, resembling a shrimp swimming at the surface of the water. It disappears and is invisible, and after a short while it reappears. The seventh is called "seething cauldron." It comes out but does not enter, just like seething hot water. All these pulse appearances indicate an extreme weakness and exhaustion of the heart; they signal that the life processes have been interrupted already. They often are part of the signs of (impending) death.

Text 11.7

2. 触诊：一般是触按胸腹和手足，如心下满症，按之坚实疼痛的为结胸，按之濡软不痛的为痞气。又如腹满拒按，按之作痛的为实为热；喜按，按之不痛的为虚为寒；腹胀叩之如鼓者为气胀，皮肤薄，按之如糟囊者为水胀。手背热为外感，手心热为阴虚；手足温者病轻，手足冷者病重；足肿按之窅然不起者为水；趺阳脉按之微细者为后天生气衰弱。

Transliteration 11.7

2. Chù-zhěn: yī-bān shì chù-àn xiōng fù hé shǒu zú, rú xīn xià mǎn-zhèng, àn zhī jiān-shí téng-tòng de wéi jié-xiōng, àn zhī rú ruǎn bù tòng de wéi pǐ-qì. Yòu rú fù-mǎn jù àn, àn zhī zuò-tòng de wéi shí wéi rè; xǐ àn, àn zhī

bù tòng de wéi xū wéi hán; fù-zhàng kòu zhī rú gǔ zhě wéi qì-zhàng, pí-fū bó, àn zhī rú zāo-náng zhě wéi shuǐ-zhàng. Shǒu-bèi rè wéi wài-gǎn, shǒu-xīn rè wéi yīn-xū; shǒu zú wēn zhě bìng qīng, shǒu zú lěng zhě bìng zhòng; zú zhǒng àn zhī yǎo rán bù qǐ zhě wéi shuǐ; fū-yáng-mài àn zhī wēi xì zhě wéi hòu-tiān shēng-qì shuāi-ruò.

Vocabulary 11.7

触按	chù-àn	touch
足	zú	foot
满症	mǎn-zhèng	fullness pathocondition
坚实	jiān-shí	hard
结胸	jié-xiōng	accumulation (of qi) in the chest
痞气	pǐ-qì	blocked qi
拒	jù	resist; refuse
作痛	zuò-tòng	cause pain
叩	kòu	knock against something
鼓	gǔ	drum
气胀	qì-zhàng	distension resulting from gas
糟	zāo	residues of fermentation
囊	náng	bag
水胀	shuǐ-zhàng	distension resulting from water
手背	shǒu-bèi	back of the hand
手心	shǒu-xīn	palm
窅	yǎo	indentation
趺	fú	instep
生气	shēng-qì	vital qi

Translation 11.7

2. Examination by touching: in general, this is the touching of chest and abdomen, as well as of hands and feet. If, for instance, in case of a fullness pathocondition below the heart, pressing (this region reveales it to be) hard and replete and painful, this is (a sign of) an accumulation (of qi) in the chest. If pressure there (shows that this region) is soft and has no pain, this is (a sign of) blocked qi. Or, if (the patient), in case of abdominal fullness, refuses to be pressed (there), and if pressing there causes pain, this is (a sign of) repletion and heat. If (the patient) welcomes pressure, and if pressing there is not painful, this is (a sign of) depletion and cold. If the abdomen is swollen, and resembles upon knocking against it a drum, this is a distension resulting from gas. If the skin is flimsy, and if under pressure it feels like a bag filled with the residues of fermentation, this is a distention resulting from water. If the back of the hand is hot, this is (a sign of) an exogenous affection; if the palm is hot, this is yin depletion. If hands and feet are warm, the illness is light; if hands and feet are cold, the illness is serious. If the feet are swollen, and if, where pressed, an indentation remains that does not rise again, this indicates water. When the yang pulse is pressed at the instep, and is felt to be feeble and fine, this indicates a weakness of vital qi of the (spleen, i.e., the) later dependence.

切脉之道，比较精微，非深入体会，不易辨别。开始临症切脉，有两点应当注意。首先，心神安定，切忌浮躁，先举，后按，再寻，举是轻手取脉，按是重手取脉，决定其浮沉，然后不轻不重寻求其形象。其次，从症候来结合脉象，是否相符，比如阳症应见阳脉，阴症应见阴脉，是为脉症符合；如果外感症而脉见细弱，或虚弱症而脉见滑大，脉症不符，预后一般不良，临症时切宜注意。

Transliteration 11.8

Qiè-mài zhī dào, bǐ-jiào jīng-wēi, fēi shēn rù tǐ-huì, bù yì biàn-bié. Kāi-shǐ lín-zhèng qiè-mài, yǒu liǎng diǎn yīng-dāng zhù-yì. Shǒu-xiān, xīn-shén ān-dìng, qiè-jì fú-zào, xiān jǔ, hòu àn, zài xún, jǔ shì qīng shǒu qǔ mài, àn shì zhòng shǒu qǔ mài, jué-dìng qí fú chén, rán-hòu bù qīng bù zhòng xún-qiú qí xíng-xiàng. Qí-cì, cóng zhèng-hòu lái jié-hé mài-xiàng, shì-fǒu xiāng-fú, bǐ-rú yáng-zhèng yīng jiàn yáng-mài, yīn-zhèng yīng jiàn yīn-mài, shì wéi mài zhèng fú-hé; rú-guǒ wài-gǎn-zhèng ér mài jiàn xì ruò, huò xū ruò zhèng ér mài jiàn huá dà, mài zhèng bù fú, yù-hòu yī-bān bù-liáng, lín-zhèng shí qiè-yí zhù-yì.

Vocabulary 11.8

道	dào	Way; doctrine; principle
精微	jīng-wēi	subtle
心神	xīn-shén	psychic constitution; mind
安定	ān-dìng	calm
切	qiè	very; certainly
切忌	qiè-jì	definitely not do/be something
浮躁	fú-zào	impatient
寻	xún	search
然后	rán-hòu	then; afterwards
符	fú	belong together
相符	xiāng-fú	correspond to each other
外感症	wài-gǎn-zhèng	pathocondition resulting from exogenous affection
切宜	qiè-yí	it is necessary

Translation 11.8

The principles of pulse-feeling are relatively subtle; without achieving a thorough understanding, it will not be easy to distinguish (the pulses). At the beginning of pulse-feeling in a clinical setting (a therapist) should pay attention to two points. First, his/her mind should be calm, and he/she must not be impatient. At the beginning is the lifting, then comes the pressure, and finally there is the search. "Lifting" is to take the pulse with a light hand. "Pressure" is to take the pulse with a heavy hand. (Thereby the therapist) determines whether (the pulse) is at the surface or deep. Then he/she searches for the shape of the (pulse with a hand that is) neither light nor heavy. Second, the pathoconditions and their signs are to be brought together with the appearance of the pulse to see whether they correspond to each other or not. For example, in case of a yang pathocondition a yang pulse should appear; in case of a yin pathocondition a yin pulse should appear. These are (examples of) pulse pathocondition correspondence. If in case of a pathocondition (resulting from) exogenous affection a fine and weak pulse appears, or if in case of a pathocondition of depletion and weakness the pulse noticed is smooth and large, then pulse and pathocondition do not correspond, and prognosis in general is bad. In clinical practice (such cases) deserve particular attention.

LESSON 12: THERAPEUTIC PRINCIPLES (I)

Text 12.1

中医治病从整体出发，十分重视病人的体力，正气，和发病的原因，邪气，把疾病看成是一个邪正相搏的过程。当邪气退却，正气进入恢复的阶段，这一斗争才算结束。也就是，正气战胜了，疾病便痊愈；邪气战胜了，就会导致病重和死亡。所以内经提出了一个纲领："虚则补之，实则泻之"。补是扶持正气的不足，泻是驱除邪气的侵害；补泻之中又有各种方法，但目的只是一个，恢复健康而已。针对着虚就用补，实就用泻，虚实同时存在，就考虑先补后泻；先泻后补；或补泻兼施。凡是从正面进行治疗，使用与病情相反性质的一种治法，不论补或泻，都叫"正治"。相反地，使用与病情性质相一致的治法，则称为"反治"。

Transliteration 12.1

Zhōng-yī zhì bìng cóng zhěng-tǐ chū-fā, shí-fēn zhòng-shì bìng-rén de tǐ-lì, zhèng-qì, hé fā-bìng de yuán-yīn, xié-qì, bǎ jí-bìng kàn-chéng shì yī gè xié zhèng xiāng bó de guò-chéng. Dāng xié-qì tuì-què, zhèng-qì jìn-rù huī-fù de jiē-duàn, zhè yī dòu-zhēng cái suàn jié-shù. Yě-jiù-shì, zhèng-qì zhàn-shèng le, jí-bìng biàn quán-yù; xié-qì zhàn-shèng le, jiù huì dǎo-zhì bìng zhòng hé sǐ-wáng. Suǒ-yǐ nèi-jīng tí-chū le yī ge gāng-lǐng: "Xū zé bǔ zhī, shí zé xiè zhī. "Bǔ shì fú-chí zhèng-qì de bù-zú, xiè shì qū-chú xié-qì de qīn-hài; bǔ-xiè zhī zhōng yòu yǒu gè zhǒng fāng-fǎ, dàn mù-dì zhǐ shì yī ge, huī-fù jiàn-kāng ér-yǐ.

Zhēn-duì zhe xū jiù yòng bǔ, shí jiù yòng xiè, xū shí tóng-shí cún-zài, jiù kǎo-lǜ xiān bǔ hòu xiè, xiān xiè hòu bǔ; huò bǔ xiè jiān-shī. Fán-shì cóng zhèng-miàn jìn-xíng zhì-liáo, shǐ-yòng yǔ bìng-qíng xiāng-fǎn xìng-zhì de yī zhǒng zhì-fǎ, bù-lùn bǔ huò xiè, dōu jiào "zhèng-zhì." Xiāng-fǎn de, shǐ-yòng yǔ bìng-qíng xìng-zhì xiāng yī-zhì de zhì-fǎ, zé chēng-wéi "fǎn-zhì."

Vocabulary 12.1

出发	chū-fā	proceed from
十分	shí-fēn	maximum
看成	kàn-chéng	view as
搏	bó	struggle
算	suàn	consider; consider as
结束	jié-shù	finish; be finished
战胜	zhàn-shèng	be victorious
导致	dǎo-zhì	lead to
死亡	sǐ-wáng	die
扶持	fú-chí	support
驱除	qū-chú	eliminate
而已	ér-yǐ	lit.: "and thereby ending" (particle indicating the close of an argument: "that's it;" often used in the sense of: "and nothing else;" "that's all")
针对	zhēn-duì	focus on
兼施	jiān-shī	apply simultaneously
凡是	fán-shì	whenever
正面	zhèng-miàn	front side; frontal
使用	shǐ-yòng	apply
正治	zhèng-zhì	direct treatment
反治	fǎn-zhì	paradoxical treatment

Translation 12.1

In treating an illness Chinese medicine proceeds from (viewing the body as an) organic whole; it pays maximum attention to the patient's bodily strength, (i.e., his/her) proper qi, and to the causes underlying the emergence of illness, (i.e.,) the evil qi, and it views an illness as a process of mutual struggle between evil and proper (qi). This fight is considered finished only at a state when the evil qi retreats while the proper qi approaches restoration. That is, when the proper qi has gained the victory, the illness is healed; when the evil qi has gained the victory, this can cause the illness to become serious and (the patient) to die. Hence the *Neijing* advanced the principle: "Depleted, supplement it; replete, drain it". To supplement means to support an insufficiency of proper qi; to drain is to eliminate an encroachment by evil qi. Within (the framework) of supplementation and draining there are all kinds of additional patterns; the goal, however, is only one: to restore health.

Against depletion supplementation is employed; (in case of) repletion draining is employed. When depletion and repletion exist at the same time, (a therapist must) consider whether to supplement first and to drain afterwards, whether to drain first and to supplement afterwards, or whether to apply supplementation and draining simultaneously. Whenever (he/she) conducts a frontal treatment, applying a therapy the nature of which is opposed to the character of the illness, this is called a "direct treatment," regardless of whether it is a supplementation or draining. Conversely, if a therapy is employed the nature of which is identical with that of the illness, this is called "paradoxical treatment."

具体的说，正治法就是寒症用热药，热症用寒药；又如症现干燥的用滋润法，拘急的用舒缓法，耗散的用收敛法。反治的用处比较少。其实反治并非真正顺从病情来治疗，表面上治法的目的似与病情同一方向，细究之，与病因仍然是相反的。例如虚性胀满症之属于消化机能迟钝的，给予补剂，而不予理气消导药，这是因为病由虚症引起，不加强其机能无从改善其症状。还有疾病严重时往往出现假象，如寒盛的格阳于外，发现烦躁不安的现象，倘以凉药治其烦躁是增加其病根，但直接用大热之药又将格阻不受，此时可以用热药凉饮方法，或在热药内加上少许凉药。这些都属反治范围，但实质上仍是正治。

Transliteration 12.2

Jù-tǐ de shuō, zhèng-zhì-fǎ jiù-shì hán-zhèng yòng rè-yào, rè-zhèng yòng hán-yào; yòu rú zhèng xiàn gān-zào de yòng zī-rùn-fǎ, jū-jí de yòng shū-huǎn-fǎ, hào-sàn de yòng shōu-liǎn-fǎ. Fǎn-zhì de yòng-chu bǐ-jiào shǎo. Qí shí fǎn-zhì bìng fēi zhēn-zhèng shùn-cóng bìng-qíng lái zhì-liáo, biǎo-miàn-shàng zhì-fǎ de mù-dì sì yǔ bìng-qíng tóng-yī fāng-xiàng, xì-jiū zhī, yǔ bìng-yīn réng-rán shì xiāng-fǎn de. Lì-rú xū xìng zhàng-mǎn zhèng zhī shǔ-yú xiāo-huà jī-néng chí-dùn de, jǐ-yǔ bǔ-jì, ér bù yǔ lǐ-qì xiāo-dǎo yào, zhè shì yīn-wèi bìng yóu xū-zhèng yǐn-qǐ, bù jiā-qiáng qí jī-néng wú cóng gǎi-shàn qí zhèng-zhuàng. Hái-yǒu jí-bìng yán-zhòng shí wǎng-wǎng chū-xiàn jiǎ-xiàng, rú hán shèng de gé-yáng-yú-wài, fā-xiàn fán-zào bù-ān de xiàn-xiàng, tǎng yǐ liáng-yào zhì qí fán-zào shì zēng-jiā qí bìng-gēn, dàn zhí-jiē yòng dà rè zhī yào yòu jiāng gé-zǔ bù shòu, cǐ shí kě-yǐ yòng rè-yào liáng yǐn fāng-fǎ, huò zài rè-yào nèi jiā-shàng shǎo-xǔ liáng-yào. Zhè-xiē dōu shǔ fǎn-zhì fàn-wéi, dàn shí-zhì-shàng réng shì zhèng-zhì.

Vocabulary 12.2

正治法	zhèng-zhì-fǎ	pattern of a direct therapy
热药	rè-yào	hot drugs
寒药	hán-yào	cold drugs
滋润法	zī-rùn-fǎ	moistening (therapy) pattern
拘急	jū-jí	tension
舒缓法	shū-huǎn-fǎ	relaxing (therapy) pattern
耗散	hào-sàn	dispersion
收敛法	shōu-liǎn-fǎ	contracting (therapy) pattern
用处	yòng-chu	application
真正	zhēn-zhèng	true; indeed; really
顺从	shùn-cóng	go along with
表面上	biǎo-miàn-shàng	on the surface
方向	fāng-xiàng	orientation
细究	xì-jiū	examine closely; look (at something) closely
仍然	réng-rán	nevertheless; still
迟钝	chí-dùn	retarded
给予	jǐ-yǔ	provide
补剂	bǔ-jì	supplementing remedy
予	yǔ	give
消导	xiāo-dǎo	digestion and transportation
无从	wú cóng	have no basis from which (to do something)
假象	jiǎ-xiàng	false phenomena
格阳于外	gé-yáng-yú-wài	repelled yang (i.e., misleading heat in the outside in case of severe cold in the interior of the body)
安	ān	quiet; peaceful
凉药	liáng-yào	cooling drugs
病根	bìng-gēn	root of an illness
格阻	gé-zǔ	barricade
加上	jiā-shàng	add

少许	shǎo-xǔ	a little; small amount
实质上	shí-zhì-shàng	in essence; in reality

Translation 12.2

In concrete terms, the pattern of a direct therapy implies the use of hot drugs in case of pathoconditions of cold, and the use of cold drugs against pathoconditions of heat. Also, if a pathocondition of dryness appears, moistening patterns are employed; in case of tensions relaxing patterns are employed, and in case of dispersion contracting patterns are employed. The applications of a paradoxical treatment are relatively few. The fact is that a paradoxical treatment is by no means a therapy that does indeed go along with the nature of the illness. On the surface it looks as if the orientation of the therapy took the same direction as the nature of the illness; looking at it closely, (though, it will become clear that) it is opposed to the cause of the illness nevertheless. For example, in case of a depletion type pathocondition of distension and fullness, associated with a retardation of the digestive faculties, a supplementing remedy is given but not a remedy that regulates the qi to (aid) digestion and transportation (of food). That is, because the illness has emerged from a pathocondition of depletion, if these faculties are not strengthened, there is no basis from which to improve this pathocondition. Also, in case of serious illnesses false phenomena appear frequently. For instance, in case of a repelled yang in the exterior (caused by a state) of cold abundance (inside the body), phenomena of vexation and restlessness appear. If this vexation and restlessness were treated by means of cooling drugs, this would strengthen the root of the illness. However, if drugs of strong heat were used straight away, they would not be let in by the (yang) barricade. In such a situation the pattern of "hot drugs and cold drink" can be employed, or a small amount of cooling drugs is added to hot drugs. All these (approaches) belong to the realm of paradoxical therapies, but in essence they are direct therapies nevertheless.

于此可见，正治和反治性质是一致的，只是战术上有所不同。运用这两种不同的战术之前，了解病因和症状是最为重要的关键性问题。后人所立的许多治疗法则，多以内经为根据加以推广应用的。至于正治和反治的具体应用，即内经中也已有较详细的指示：关于病因方面的，如"寒者热之；热者寒之；客者除之；劳者温之；其实者散而泻之"，此皆为正治法；又如"寒之而热者取之阴；热之而寒者取之阳"，此皆为反治法。关于症状方面的，如"坚者削之；结者散之；留者攻之；燥者濡之；惊者平之"，此皆为正治法；又如"塞因塞用；通因通用"，此皆为反治法。

Transliteration 12.3

Yú-cǐ-kě-jiàn, zhèng-zhì hé fǎn-zhì xìng-zhì shì yī-zhì de, zhǐ shì zhàn-shù shàng yǒu suǒ bù-tóng. Yùn-yòng zhè liǎng zhǒng bù-tóng de zhàn-shù zhī qián, liǎo-jiě bìng-yīn hé zhèng-zhuàng shì zuì-wéi zhòng-yào de guān-jiàn-xìng wèn-tí. Hòu-rén suǒ lì de xǔ-duō zhì-liáo fǎ-zé, duō yǐ nèi-jīng wéi gēn-jù jiā-yǐ tuī-guǎng yīng-yòng de. Zhì-yú zhèng-zhì hé fǎn-zhì de jù-tǐ yīng-yòng, jí nèi-jīng zhōng yě yǐ yǒu jiào xiáng-xì de zhǐ-shì: guān-yú bìng-yīn fāng-miàn de, rú "hán zhě rè zhī; rè zhě hán zhī; kè zhě chú zhī; láo zhě wēn zhī; qí shí zhě sàn ér xiè zhī," cǐ jiē wéi zhèng-zhì-fǎ; yòu rú "hán zhī ér rè zhě qǔ zhī yīn; rè zhī ér hán zhě qǔ zhī yáng," cǐ jiē wéi fǎn-zhì-fǎ. Guān-yú zhèng-zhuàng fāng-miàn de, rú "jiān zhě xuē zhī; jié zhě sàn zhī; liú zhě gōng zhī; zào zhě rú zhī; jīng zhě píng zhī," cǐ jiē wéi zhèng-zhì-fǎ; yòu rú "sāi yīn sāi yòng; tōng yīn tōng yòng," cǐ jiē wéi fǎn-zhì-fǎ.

Vocabulary 12.3

于此可见	yú-cǐ-kě-jiàn	that shows; from this it can be seen
战术	zhàn-shù	tactics
战术上	zhàn-shù shàng	in tactics

有所	yǒu suǒ	there is something which; a little
了解	liǎo-jiě	find out; understand
关键性	guān-jiàn-xìng	central; essential
后人	hòu-rén	people in later times
法则	fǎ-zé	rule; law
推广	tuī-guǎng	extend
至于	zhì-yú	as for; as far as
详细	xiáng-xì	detailed
客	kè	guest; take residence
除	chú	eliminate
取	qǔ	take
之	zhī	this
反治法	fǎn-zhì-fǎ	paradox therapy pattern
削	xuē	cut
惊	jīng	tense
平	pīng	pacify
塞	sāi	obstruction
通	tōng	penetrate; make passable

Translation 12.3

From this it is obvious that the nature of direct and paradoxical therapies is identical; it is just that the tactics are not the same. Before these two different tactics are applied, the most important key issue is to find out the cause of the illness and (to determine) the pathoconditions. Many therapeutic patterns introduced by people in later times are extended applications having the *Neijing* as their basis. The *Neijing* contains relatively detailed instructions already for a concrete application of direct and paradoxical therapies. (When it states) in view of the causes of an illness "if it is cold, heat it; if it is hot, cool it; if it has taken residence, remove it; if it is exhausted, warm it; if it is replete, disperse and drain it," then these are all direct therapy patterns. Furthermore, (when it states), for example, "whenever it is cooled and heat (emerges nevertheless), take it from the yin; whenever it is heated, and cold (emerges nevertheless), take it from the yang," all these are paradoxical therapeutic patterns. In view of pathoconditions (the *Neijing*) states, for instance: "If it is hard, cut it; if it is knotted, disperse it; if it is stagnant, attack it; if it has dried, moisten it; if it is tense, relax it; if it is dispersed, contract it; if it is aroused, pacify it." All these are patterns of direct therapy. Or (when it states), for instance: "because (the illness is an) obstruction, obstructing (drugs) are employed (to treat it), because (the illness is) passage, (drugs) opening passages are employed (to treat it)," then these are all paradoxical therapeutic patterns.

Text 12.4

治本和治标也是一般常用的治疗法则，必须明白标本，才能在治疗上决定轻重，缓急，先后等措施。标本的意义有两项：

1. 从人体与疾病来说，人体是本，疾病是标。治病的目的为了病人恢复健康，如果只顾疾病，不考虑人体，势必病去而元气大伤，或元气伤而病仍留存，或带来后遗症成为残废，甚至病除而人亦随亡，这是首先应该注意的。

2. 从疾病的原因和症状来说，原因是本，症状是标。症状的发生必有一个因素，能把因素去掉，症状自然消失，中医常说"治病必求于本"，即是指此。

Transliteration 12.4

Zhì běn hé zhì biāo yě shì yī-bān cháng-yòng de zhì-liáo fǎ-zé, bì-xū míng-bái biāo-běn, cái néng zài zhì-liáo shàng jué-dìng qīng zhòng, huǎn-jí, xiān-hòu děng cuò-shī. Biāo-běn de yì-yì yǒu liǎng xiàng:

1. Cóng rén-tǐ yǔ jí-bìng lái shuō, rén-tǐ shì běn, jí-bìng shì biāo. Zhì-bìng de mù-dì wéi-le bìng-rén huī-fù jiàn-kāng, rú-guǒ zhǐ gù jí-bìng, bù kǎo-lǜ rén-tǐ, shì-bì bìng qù ér yuán-qì dà shāng, huò yuán-qì shāng ér bìng réng liú-cún, huò dài-lái hòu-yí-zhèng chéng-wéi cán-fèi, shèn-zhì bìng chú ér rén yì suí wáng, zhè shì shǒu-xiān yīng-gāi zhù-yì de.

2. Cóng jí-bìng de yuán-yīn hé zhèng-zhuàng lái shuō, yuán-yīn shì běn, zhèng-zhuàng shì biāo. Zhèng-zhuàng de fā-shēng bì yǒu yī ge yīn-sù, néng bǎ yīn-sù qù-diào, zhèng-zhuàng zì-rán xiāo-shī, zhōng-yī cháng shuō "zhì bìng bì qiú yú běn," jí shì zhǐ cǐ.

Vocabulary 12.4

标	biāo	tip
标本	biāo-běn	tip and root
先后	xiān hòu	earlier and later
措施	cuò-shī	measure; approach

势必	shì-bì	inevitable
留存	liú-cún	stay
带来	dài-lái	cause; lead to
后遗症	hòu-yí-zhèng	sequelae (of an illness)
残废	cán-fèi	permanent disablement
随	suí	follow; afterwards; subsequently
去掉	qù-diào	eliminate
消失	xiāo-shī	vanish
求	qiú	search

Translation 12.4

To treat the root and to treat the tip are two further frequently employed therapeutic patterns. (A therapist) must understand (the meaning of) tip and root, and is only then able to determine, in a treatment, light and heavy, slow and fast, as well as earlier and later measures. The meaning of tip and root is twofold:

1. As far as the human body and (its) illnesses are concerned, the human body is the root, and the illness is the tip. It is the objective of the treatment of an illness to restore the patient's health. If (a therapist) is concerned with the illness only, and fails to take into account the body, the inevitable result will be that the illness is eliminated and the original qi receives great harm, or the original qi is harmed, and the illness stays nevertheless, or (the treatment) causes sequelae leading to permanent disablement. This may even go so far that the illness may be eliminated and that person subsequently perishes too. This should be paid attention to first.

2. In terms of causes and pathoconditions of illnesses, the causes are the roots, and the pathoconditions are the tips. Any emergence of a pathocondition must have a causal factor; if the causal factor can be eliminated, the pathoconditions will vanish as a matter of course. In Chinese medicine it is often stated: "To treat an illness it is necessary to search for its root." That refers exactly to this (approach).

本就是根本，根源，治病必须重视根本，找寻根源，了解其所以然。也就是治病必须抓住主要的，主要的解决了，次要的自然迎刃而解。因而有祛邪扶正和扶正祛邪两种说法，认为扶正则邪自却，邪却则正自复。这两种说法表面上似有矛盾，其实都是从根本上出发，因虚而致病自以扶正为主，因邪而致病自以祛邪为先。意思是吐痰，失血，无汗，发热，气喘，遗精等均属表面的现象，酿成这类病症各有主要的原因，不探本寻源想办法，仅用化痰，止血，发汗，清热，平喘，固精等常法是不起作用的。

Transliteration 12.5

Běn jiù-shì gēn-běn, gēn-yuán, zhì bìng bì-xū zhòng-shì gēn-běn, zhǎo-xún gēn-yuán, liǎo-jiě qí suǒ-yǐ rán. Yě-jiù-shì zhì bìng bì-xū zhuā-zhù zhǔ-yào de, zhǔ-yào de jiě-jué le, cì-yào de zì-rán yíng-rèn-ér-jiě. Yīn-ér yǒu qū xié fú zhèng hé fú zhèng qū xié liǎng zhǒng shuō-fǎ, rèn-wéi fú zhèng zé xié zì què, xié què zé zhèng zì fù. Zhè liǎng zhǒng shuō-fǎ biǎo-miàn-shàng sì yǒu máo-dùn, qí-shí dōu-shì cóng gēn-běn shàng chū-fā, yīn xū ér zhì bìng zì yǐ fú-zhèng wéi zhǔ, yīn xié ér zhì bìng zì yǐ qū-xié wéi xiān. Yì-sì shì tǔ-tán, shī-xuè, wú-hàn, fā-rè, qì-chuǎn, yí-jīng děng jūn shǔ biǎo-miàn de xiàn-xiàng, niàng-chéng zhè-lèi bìng-zhèng gè yǒu zhǔ-yào de yuán-yīn, bù tàn běn xún yuán xiǎng bàn-fǎ, jǐn yòng huà-tán, zhǐ-xuè, fā-hàn, qīng-rè, píng-chuǎn, gù-jīng děng cháng-fǎ shì bù qǐ zuò-yòng de.

Vocabulary 12.5

根本	gēn-běn	basic root
根源	gēn-yuán	basic source
找寻	zhǎo-xún	search
抓住	zhuā-zhù	get a hold of
解决	jiě-jué	resolve
次要	cì-yào	of secondary importance
迎刃而解	yíng-rèn-ér-jiě	solve easily
扶	fú	support
却	què	retreat; leave

复	fù	return
矛盾	máo-dùn	contradiction
自	zì	of course
扶正	fú-zhèng	support the proper
祛邪	qū-xié	eliminate the evil
吐痰	tǔ-tán	vomit phlegm
表面上	biǎo-miàn-shàng	outside
探	tàn	investigate
想	xiǎng	think of; consider
办法	bàn-fǎ	measure; method
化痰	huà-tán	transform phlegm
止血	zhǐ-xuè	stop bleeding
平喘	píng-chuǎn	calm panting
固精	gù-jīng	stabilize semen
常法	cháng-fǎ	common pattern

Translation 12.5

Root stands for basic root, basic source. In treating an illness it is necessary to pay attention to its basic root, and search for its basic source, to understand why it is as it is. That is, in treating an illness it is necessary to get a hold of the principal (issue); once the principal (issue) is resolved, (all issues of) secondary importance will be solved easily. Hence there are the two sayings of "eliminate the evil and support the proper" and "support the proper and eliminate the evil." (They are based on) the assumption that if the proper is supported, the evil will leave by itself, and once the evil has left, the proper will return by itself. On the surface, these two sayings appear to be contradictory; the fact is that they both proceed from the basic root (of an illness). If an illness has arisen because of a depletion, to support the proper (qi) will be the major (approach); if the illness has arisen because of (an intrusion of) evil (qi), eliminating the evil (qi) will be the primary (task). That means, to vomit phlegm, loss of blood, failure to sweat, fever, panting, or involuntary emissions, all these are outside phenomena, and there are major causes creating each of these pathoconditions. If measures (to treat these pathoconditions) are considered without investigating their roots and (without) searching for their sources, and if merely common patterns are employed that transform phlegm, stop the bleeding, induce sweating, cool heat, calm the panting, stabilize the semen, and so on, then these will be of no use.

Text 12.6

虽然，治病必须求本，但也不能忽视其标。我们体会求因当然是必要的，辨症也同样重要，辨症就是为了求因。但在另一方面，求得主因之外还要求得主症，因为迅速的缓和症状，也是解除病人痛苦的重要一环。例如感冒风寒，发热头痛，浑身酸楚，手足无措。风寒是主因，其它都是由风寒引起的症状，但在症状中发热是一个主症，热度的高低能使其它症状加剧和轻减。所以用发汗法来疏散风寒是主要治法，但加入一些清解药来帮助退热，以减轻其它症状，也是合理的。前人治病有单从原因用药的，也有兼顾症状的。

Transliteration 12.6

Suī-rán, zhì bìng bì-xū qiú běn, dàn yě bù néng hū-shì qí biāo. Wǒ-men tǐ-huì qiú yīn dāng-rán shì bì-yào de, biàn-zhèng yě tóng-yàng zhòng-yào, biàn-zhèng jiù-shì wéi-le qiú yīn. Dàn zài lìng-yī fāng-miàn, qiú-de zhǔ-yīn zhī-wài hái yào qiú-de zhǔ-zhèng, yīn-wèi xùn-sù de huǎn-hé zhèng-zhuàng, yě shì jiě-chú bìng-rén tòng-kǔ de zhòng-yào yī huán. Lì-rú gǎn-mào fēng-hán, fā-rè tóu-tòng, hún-shēn suān-chǔ, shǒu zú wú cuò. Fēng-hán shì zhǔ-yīn, qí-tā dōu-shì yóu fēng-hán yǐn-qǐ de zhèng-zhuàng, dàn zài zhèng-zhuàng zhōng fā-rè shì yī ge zhǔ-zhèng, rè-dù de gāo-dī néng shǐ qí-tā zhèng-zhuàng jiā-jù hé qīng-jiǎn. Suǒ-yǐ yòng fā-hàn-fǎ lái shū-sàn fēng-hán shì zhǔ-yào zhì-fǎ, dàn jiā-rù yī-xiē qīng-jiě-yào lái bāng-zhù tuì rè, yǐ jiǎn-qīng qí-tā zhèng-zhuàng, yě shì hé-lǐ de. Qián-rén zhì bìng yǒu dān cóng yuán-yīn yòng yào de, yě yǒu jiān-gù zhèng-zhuàng de.

Vocabulary 12.6

忽视	hū-shì	neglect; ignore
我们	wǒ-men	we
迅速	xùn-sù	speedy
缓和	huǎn-hé	alleviate
浑身	hún-shēn	the entire body
酸楚	suān-chǔ	ache
措	cuò	make use of
热度	rè-dù	degree of fever

加剧	jiā-jù	increase
轻减	qīng-jiǎn	lessen
清解药	qīng-jiě-yào	cooling drugs
减轻	jiǎn-qīng	alleviate
合理	hé-lǐ	be appropriate

Translation 12.6

Even though, when treating illnesses, it is essential to search for their roots, their tips must not be neglected either. We know from experience that searching for the cause (of an illness) is of course essential; to differentiate pathoconditions is equally important. After all, to differentiate pathoconditions serves to search for the cause (of an illness). On the other hand, though, in addition to finding out the main cause, the main pathocondition should be identified because a speedy alleviation of the pathoconditions is also an important element in the elimination of the patient's suffering. For example, in case of a common cold (caused by) wind cold, (the patient) develops fever and has headache. The entire body aches, and (the patient) cannot make use of his/her hands or feet. The wind cold is the major cause, and all the other (problems) are pathoconditions provoked by wind cold. However, among the pathoconditions, the fever is the main pathocondition; and the degree of the fever may cause the other pathoconditions to increase or lessen in severity. Hence the major therapy is to apply a sudorific pattern to disperse the wind cold. However, it is also appropriate to add some cooling drugs to support the removal of the heat, and this way to alleviate the other pathoconditions. When the people in former times treated illnesses, there were (occasions when) they applied drugs solely proceeding from the cause, and there were other (situations when) they took the pathoconditions into account too.

临症上如果认为标症已占重要位置时，应当采取先治其标的方法。例如：因肝病引起的腹水症，肝病是本，腹水是标。但已到腹部胀满，呼吸困难，二便不利的地步，如同洪水泛滥，不予疏浚，无法救其危急。此时再不能用疏肝和肝，只有峻剂泻水，俟水退后再商治本。又如：小便不利能很快促使病情恶化，任何疾病发现小便不利时，即当以通利小便为急。前人说"急则治标"，治标原是一种权宜之计，达到目的以后，就不宜继续使用。

Transliteration 12.7

Lín-zhèng shàng rú-guǒ rèn-wéi biāo-zhèng yǐ zhàn zhòng-yào wèi-zhì shí, yīng-dāng cǎi-qǔ xiān zhì qí biāo de fāng-fǎ. Lì-rú: yīn gān-bìng yǐn-qǐ de fù-shuǐ zhèng, gān-bìng shì běn, fù-shuǐ shì biāo. Dàn yǐ dào fù-bù, zhàng-mǎn, hū-xī kùn-nán, èr-biàn bù-lì de dì-bù, rú-tóng hóng-shuǐ fàn-làn, bù-yǔ shū-jùn, wú fǎ jiù qí wēi-jí. Cǐ-shí zài bù néng yòng shū-gān hé-gān, zhǐ yǒu jùn jì xiè shuǐ, sì shuǐ tuì hòu zài shāng zhì-běn. Yòu-rú: xiǎo-biàn bù-lì néng hěn kuài cù-shǐ bìng-qíng è-huà, rèn-hé jí-bìng fā-xiàn xiǎo-biàn bù-lì shí, jí dāng yǐ tōng-lì xiǎo-biàn wéi jí. Qián-rén shuō "jí zé zhì-biāo," zhì-biāo yuán-shì yī zhǒng quán-yí-zhī-jì, dá-dào mù-dì yǐ-hòu, jiù bù-yí jì-xù shǐ-yòng.

Vocabulary 12.7

标症	biāo-zhèng	tip pathocondition
占	zhàn	assume (a stage)
腹水	fù-shuǐ	abdominal water
腹部	fù-bù	abdominal section
地步	dì-bù	condition; stage
如同	rú-tóng	equal to; as if
洪水	hóng-shuǐ	flood; flood water
泛滥	fàn-làn	inundation
不予	bù-yǔ	not to grant
疏浚	shū-jùn	dredge
救	jiù	rescue
危急	wēi-jí	critical; in severe danger
和肝	hé-gān	harmonize the liver
峻	jùn	drastic
俟	sì	wait; only then
商	shāng	consider
治本	zhì-běn	treat the root (of an illness)
促使	cù-shǐ	lead to
恶化	è-huà	aggravate; aggravation

治标	zhì-biāo	treat the tip (of an illness)
原是	yuán-shì	is/are basically
权宜之计	quán-yí-zhī-jì	expediency
达到	dá-dào	attain; reach
达到...以后	dá-dào ... yǐ-hòu	after ... has been attained
不宜	bù-yí	should not
继续	jì-xù	continue

Translation 12.7

If the conclusion has been reached, in clinical practice, that a tip pathocondition has assumed a critical stage already, it is necessary to select a pattern to treat this tip first. For example, in case of a pathocondition of abdominal water provoked by a liver illness, the liver illness is the root, and the abdominal water is the tip. However, if (the patient) has reached a condition where the abdominal section is distended and full, where breathing is difficult, and where the urine and the stools do not pass freely, this is as if flood water has caused inundation. If (the water is) not led away by digging (a channel), there will be no way to rescue (the patient) from the ensuing danger. At this moment (drugs) to sooth the liver or to harmonize the liver cannot be employed. There is only (one possibility, i.e.,) to drain the water with drastic remedies, and only after the water has been removed (the therapist may) consider further how to treat the root (of the illness). Or another example: When the urine does not pass, this may lead within a very short time to an aggravation of the patient's condition. Whenever in the course of an illness anuria appears, restoring the free passage of the urine must be considered as urgent. The people in former times said: "In case of urgency, treat the tip." To treat the tip is basically an expediency; once its objective has been attained, its application should not be continued.

Text 12.8

一个人同时患两种病时，也须分别标本，一般对先病为本，后病为标。先病多指顽固性慢性疾病，后病则以感冒等时症为多，在这种情况下应当先治感冒，后治慢性病。因为慢性病不是旦夕能除，而感冒等时症容易解除，且亦能发展成为严重症候，促使慢性病的恶化。也有本来是感冒症，忽然并发胃肠病，下利清谷，脉浮转沉，则恐外邪乘虚内陷，又须急治其里，再解其标。这些又说明了治疗上以治本为原则，在这原则下还应掌握先后缓急，灵活运用。

Transliteration 12.8

Yī ge rén tóng-shí huàn liǎng zhǒng bìng shí, yě xū fēn-bié biāo-běn, yībān duì xiān-bìng wéi běn, fòu-bìng wéi biāo. Xiān-bìng duō zhǐ wán-gù-xìng màn-xìng jí-bìng, hòu-bìng zé yǐ gǎn-mào děng shí-zhèng wéi duō, zài zhè zhǒng qíng-kuàng xià yīng-dāng xiān zhì gǎn-mào, hòu zhì màn-xìng-bìng. Yīn-wéi màn-xìng-bìng bù shì dàn-xī néng chú, ér gǎn-mào děng shí-zhèng róng-yì jiě-chú, qiě yì néng fā-zhǎn chéng-wéi yán-zhòng zhèng-hòu, cù-shǐ màn-xìng-bìng de è-huà. Yě yǒu běn-lái shì gǎn-mào zhèng, hū-rán bìng fā wèi-cháng-bìng, xià-lì qīng-gǔ, mài fú zhuàn chén, zé kǒng wài-xié chéng xū nèi xiàn, yòu xū jí zhì qí lǐ, zài jiě qí biāo. Zhè-xiē yòu shuō-míng le zhì-liáo shàng yǐ zhì-běn wéi yuán-zé, zài zhè yuán-zé xià hái yīng zhǎng-wò xiān-hòu huǎn-jí, líng-huó yùn-yòng.

Vocabulary 12.8

先病	xiān-bìng	the earlier illness
后病	hòu-bìng	the later illness
顽固性	wán-gù-xìng	stubborn
慢性	màn-xìng	chronic
时症	shí-zhèng	seasonal pathocondition
慢性病	màn-xìng-bìng	chronic illness
旦夕	dàn-xī	dawn and dusk; in one day
本来	běn-lái	originally
忽然	hū-rán	all of a sudden
胃肠病	wèi-cháng-bìng	illness of stomach and intestines
陷	xiàn	sink
原则	yuán-zé	guiding principle

Translation 12.8

When one single person suffers from two kinds of illness at the same time, it is necessary too to distinguish between tips and roots. In general, the earlier illness is considered the root, while the illness that appeared later is considered the tip. "Earlier illness" often refers to stubborn, chronic illnesses; "later illnesses" are mostly seasonal pathoconditions like the common cold. Under such circumstances the common cold should be treated first, and the chronic illness afterwards. The reason is that chronic illnesses cannot be eliminated between dawn and dusk, while seasonal pathoconditions such as common cold can be removed easily. Also, (the latter) are able to develop into serious pathoconditions, quickly causing the chronic illness to aggravate. It also happens that (a patient) originally (suffered from) a pathocondition of common cold, and all of a sudden developed an illness of the stomach and of the intestines in addition, with a diarrhea of undigested food, and a pulse that is at the surface and changes into being deep. Here it is to be feared that an exogenous evil takes advantage of a depletion and sinks into the interior. Again, it is necessary (first) to quickly treat the interior and then resolve the (problem at the) tip. All these (examples) are to explain that in therapy treating the roots is considered as the guiding principle, and that on the basis of this guiding principle (a therapist) should master and flexibly apply (approaches as they appear in) earlier and later, slow and quick (treatments).

Text 13.1

确定病症后，紧接着的便是选择治疗方法。治法分发汗，催吐，攻下，和解，清凉，温热，消导和滋补等，简称为汗，吐，下，和，清，温，消，补八法。这八法针对病因，症状和发病的部位，指出了治疗的方向，在临症上灵活运用。

1. 汗法：以疏散风寒为目的，常用于外邪侵犯肌表，即内经所说"在皮者汗而发之"，故亦称解表，解肌，疏解。比如外感初起，恶寒发热，骨节痛，得汗后便热退身凉，诸症消失。汗法包括宣肺法在内，如伤风咳嗽，鼻塞，音嘎，用轻扬上焦的药，目的不在发汗，但使肺气宣通。

Transliteration 13.1

Què-dìng bìng-zhèng hòu, jǐn-jiē-zhe de biàn shì xuǎn-zé zhì-liáo fāng-fǎ. Zhì-fǎ fēn fā-hàn, cuī-tù, gōng-xià, hé-jiě, qīng-liáng, wēn-rè, suǒ-dǎo hé zī-bǔ děng, jiǎn chēng-wéi hàn, tù, xià, hé, qīng, wēn, xiāo, bǔ bā fǎ. Zhè bā fǎ zhēn-duì bìng-yīn, zhèng-zhuàng hé fā-bìng de bù-wèi, zhǐ chū le zhì-liáo de fāng-xiàng, zài lín-zhèng shàng líng-huó yùn-yòng.

1. Hàn-fǎ: yǐ shū-sàn fēng-hán wéi mù-dì, cháng-yòng yú wài-xié qīn-fàn jī-biǎo, jí nèi-jīng suǒ shuō “zài pí zhě hàn ér fā zhī,” gù yì chēng jiě-biǎo, jiě-jī, shū-jiě. Bǐ-rú wài-gǎn chū-qǐ, wù-hán fā-rè, gǔ-jié-tòng, dé hàn hòu biàn rè tuì shēn liáng, zhū zhèng xiāo-shī.

Hàn-fǎ bāo-kuò xuān-fèi-fǎ zài nèi, rú shāng-fēng ké-sòu, bí-sè, yīn-gā, yòng qīng-yáng shàng-jiāo de yào, mù-dì bù zài fā-hàn, dàn shǐ fèi-qì xuān-tōng.

Vocabulary 13.1

紧接	jǐn-jiē	follow next
选择	xuǎn-zé	select

催吐	cuī-tù	induced vomiting
攻下	gōng-xià	offensive purgation
和解	hé-jiě	harmonization and resolution
清凉	qīng-liáng	cool
温热	wēn-rè	warm and heat
滋补	zī-bǔ	nourish and supplement
简	jiǎn	short (in the sense of uncomplicated)
八法	bā-fǎ	the eight patterns
肌表	jī-biǎo	muscular exterior
解肌	jiě-jī	resolve the muscles
疏解	shū-jiě	course and open
骨节痛	gǔ-jié-tòng	bone and joint pain
宣肺法	xuān-fèi-fǎ	pattern of transmitting the lung (qi)
音嘎	yīn-gā	hoarse voice
轻扬	qīng-yáng	lift
宣通	xuān-tōng	promote an unimpeded flow

Translation 13.1

After illness and pathoconditions have been identified, the next step is to select a therapeutic pattern. Among the therapeutic patterns distinction is made between effusing sweat, induced vomiting, offensive purgation, harmonization and resolution, dissolving and guiding, as well as nourishing and supplementing; in short these are called the eight patterns of sweating, vomiting, purging, harmonizing, cooling, warming, dissolving, and supplementing. These eight patterns are directed against the causes of an illness, the pathoconditions, or the location where an illness has developed, and they indicate the direction of the therapy. In clinical reality they are employed flexibly.

1. The pattern of sweating: It has as its objective the dispersion of wind cold. It is used regularly against external evils having invaded the muscular

exterior. This is just what is stated in the *Neijing*: "When it is in the skin, effuse it through sweating." Hence (this pattern) is also called: "to open the outside," "to open the muscles" or "to course and open." For example, when an exogenous affection first emerges, (the patient) has an aversion to cold and develops heat. The bones and the joints ache. After a sweating, the heat will retreat, and the body cools down. All pathoconditions disappear.

The pattern of sweating includes also the pattern of transmitting the lung (qi). For instance, when in case of harm caused by wind, (accompanied by) coughing, nasal congestion, and a hoarse voice, drugs are used exerting a lifting effect on the upper burner,[1] the objective is not to induce sweating but to promote the unimpeded flow of the lung qi.

Note

1 In this statement, the term "upper burner" is used in the meaning of "heart and lung," and refers here specifically to the lung. Cf. Text 5.7.

2.吐法：常用于咽喉，胸膈痰食堵塞。如喉症中的缠喉症，锁喉症皆为风痰郁火壅塞，胀闭难忍；又如积食停滞，胸膈饱满疼痛，只要上涌倾出，故亦称涌吐。吐法都用催吐药，但亦有因症用药，服药后用鸡毛或手指探喉使其恶出，所以又有探吐之称。吐法多用在胃上部有形的实邪，一般多是一吐为快，不须反复使用。某些病人先有呕吐的，不但不可再吐，还要防其伤胃，给予和中方法。其他，凡虚弱的病体或新产后，严重的脚气以及四肢厥冷的，均不宜用吐。

Transliteration 13.2

2. Tù-fǎ: cháng-yòng yú yān-hóu, xiōng gé tán shí dǔ-sè. Rú hóu-zhèng zhōng de chán-hóu-zhèng, suǒ-hóu-zhèng jiē wéi fēng-tán yù-huǒ yōng-sè, zhàng bì nán rěn; yòu-rú jī-shí tíng-zhì, xiōng gé bǎo-mǎn téng-tòng, zhǐ yào shàng-yǒng qīng chū, gù yì chēng yǒng-tù.

Tù-fǎ dōu yòng cuī-tù-yào, dàn yì yǒu yīn zhèng yòng yào, fú-yào hòu yòng jī-máo huò shǒu-zhǐ tàn hóu shǐ qí è chū, suǒ-yǐ yòu yǒu tàn-tù zhī chēng.

Tù-fǎ duō yòng zài wèi shàng bù yǒu-xíng de shí-xié, yī-bān duō shì yī tù wéi kuài, bù xū fǎn-fù shǐ-yòng. Mǒu-xiē bìng-rén xiān yǒu ǒu-tù de, bù-dàn bù-kě zài tù, hái yào fáng qí shāng wèi, jǐ-yǔ hé-zhōng-fāng-fǎ. Qí-tā, fán xū-ruò de bìng-tǐ huò xīn chǎn hòu, yán-zhòng de jiǎo-qì yǐ-jí sì-zhī jué-lěng de, jūn bù-yí yòng tù.

Vocabulary 13.2

吐法	tù-fǎ	the pattern of (induced) vomiting
堵塞	dǔ-sè	block
喉症	hóu-zhèng	pathoconditions (affecting) the throat
缠喉症	chán-hóu-zhèng	pathocondition of "strangled throat"

锁喉症	suǒ-hóu-zhèng	pathocondition of "obstructed throat"
郁火	yù-huǒ	depressed fire
壅塞	yōng-sè	blockage
闭	bì	closure
忍	rěn	bear; endure
积食	jī-shí	food accumulation
饱满	bǎo-mǎn	(feeling of) fullness
只要	zhǐ-yào	all that is necessary is
上涌	shàng-yǒng	gush upwards
倾	qīng	tip up; overturn; pour out
涌吐	yǒng-tù	ejection through vomiting
催吐药	cuī-tù-yào	drugs inducing vomiting; emetic drugs
服药	fú-yào	take drugs
鸡毛	jī-máo	a chicken's feather
手指	shǒu-zhǐ	finger
恶	è	bad
探吐	tàn-tù	vomiting (induced) by poking (into the throat)
实邪	shí-xié	solid evil
快	kuài	wellbeing
某些	mǒu-xiē	certain (people, things, etc.)
不但	bù-dàn	not only
和中方法	hé-zhōng-fāng-fǎ	pattern to harmonize the center
病体	bìng-tǐ	physical condition during an illness
脚气	jiǎo-qì	beriberi

Translation 13.2

2. The pattern of (induced) vomiting: It is regularly used when the throat, or the chest and the diaphragm, are blocked by phlegm or food. For example, among the pathoconditions (affecting) the throat, the

pathoconditions of "strangled throat" and "obstructed throat" are both blockages (caused by) wind phlegm or depressed fire;[1] (they are accompanied by) distension and closure, and are hard to bear. Or, in case of blockages resulting from food accumulations, when (the region of) chest and diaphragm (experiences a feeling of) fullness and pain, all that is necessary is to eject (the food or the phlegm) upwards and (make it) leave (the body as if it was) poured out. Hence this is called "ejection through vomiting."

The pattern of (induced) vomiting always employs emetic drugs. However, it may also be that drugs are used in accordance with the pathoconditions, and that after taking the drugs (the patient) takes recourse to a chicken's feather or to a finger to poke into the throat and cause the bad to come out. Hence there is also the term "(induced) vomiting by poking (into the throat)."

The pattern of (induced) vomiting is often used in case of tangible, solid evil situated in the upper part of the stomach. In general, one (application of induced) vomiting restores the (patient's) wellbeing; it is inappropriate to employ (this approach) repeatedly. Certain patients who have vomited already, they not only must not (be stimulated to) vomit again, they also require that their stomach is protected from harm and that a (therapeutic) pattern is applied to harmonize their center. Furthermore, in all situations where (the patient) has a weak physical constitution, or has just had a delivery, (suffers from) severe beriberi, or if his/her four limbs are cold because of recession (of yang qi), it is inappropriate to resort to (induced) vomiting.

Note

1 "Depressed fire" stands for "depressed yang qi."

3. 下法：一般多指通大便，用来排除肠内宿粪积滞，故也称攻下，泻下。攻下剂分为两类，一种是峻下，用猛烈泻下药，大多用于实热症有津涸阴亡的趋势时。一种是缓下，又分两类，一类是用较为缓和的泻药，一类是用油润之剂帮助下达。但不论峻下或缓下，都宜于里实症，这是一致的。由于里实的原因不同，又分凉下和温下二种。凉下是指苦寒性质的泻剂，温下是指辛热性质的泻剂。一般应用以苦寒为多，因多数便闭或下利症，由于热结或湿热引起。

Transliteration 13.3

3. Xià-fǎ: yī-bān duō zhǐ tōng dà-biàn, yòng lái pái-chú cháng nèi sù-fèn jī-zhì, gù yě chēng gōng-xià, xiè-xià.

Gōng-xià-jì fēn-wéi liǎng lèi, yī zhǒng shì jùn-xià, yòng měng-liè xiè-xià-yào, dà-duō yòng yú shí-rè-zhèng yǒu jīn hé yīn wáng de qū-shì shí. Yī zhǒng shì huǎn-xià, yòu fēn liǎng lèi, yī lèi shì yòng jiào wéi huǎn-hé de xiè-yào, yī lèi shì yòng yóu rùn zhī jì bāng-zhù xià-dá. Dàn bù-lùn jùn-xià huò huǎn-xià, dōu yí yú lǐ-shí-zhèng, zhè shì yī-zhì de.

Yóu-yú lǐ-shí de yuán-yīn bù-tóng, yòu fēn liáng-xià hé wēn-xià èr zhǒng. Liáng-xià shì zhǐ kǔ hán xìng-zhì de xiè-jì, wēn-xià shì zhǐ xīn rè xìng-zhì de xiè-jì. Yī-bān yīng-yòng yǐ kǔ hán wéi duō, yīn duō shù biàn-bì huò xià-lì zhèng, yóu-yú rè-jié huò shī-rè yǐn-qǐ.

Vocabulary 13.3

宿粪	sù-fèn	faeces staying (in the intestines)
积滞	jī-zhì	accumulation blockages
泻下	xiè-xià	draining purgation
攻下剂	gōng-xià-jì	remedies for a charge downwards
峻下	jùn-xià	drastic purgation
猛烈	měng-liè	violent
泻下药	xiè-xià-yào	drugs for draining downwards
实热症	shí-rè-zhèng	pathoconditions of repletion heat

涸	hé	dry up
趋势	qū-shì	tend; tendency
缓下	huǎn-xià	mild purging
泻药	xiè-yào	draining drugs
下达	xià-dá	defecation
里实	lǐ-shí	internal repletion
里实症	lǐ-shí-zhèng	pathoconditions of internal repletion
热结	rè-jié	heat accumulations

Translation 13.3

3. The pattern of purgation: In general (this approach) refers to clearing the passage of stools. It is applied to remove accumulation blockages of faeces staying in the intestines. Hence (this approach) is also called "forced purgation," or "draining purgation."

The remedies for an offensive purgation are divided into two types. One type is (used for) drastic purgation; it relies on drugs violently draining downwards. It is used mostly in cases of pathoconditions of repletion heat when the fluids tend to dry up, and the yin qi is about to vanish. The other type is for mild purging; it is divided into two types again. One type includes an application of relatively mild draining drugs; the other type includes an application of oiling and moistening remedies to aid defecation. However, both drastic purgation and mild purgation are suitable for pathoconditions of internal repletion; in this regard there is no difference.

Because the causes of internal repletion may differ, (Chinese medicine) further distinguishes between the two types of cooling purgation and warming purgation. Cooling purgation refers to draining remedies of a bitter and cold nature; warming purgation refers to draining remedies of an acrid and hot nature. Generally speaking, bitter and cold (remedies) are used more often because the majority of the pathoconditions of constipation or diarrhea are caused by heat accumulations or damp heat.

4.和法：和是和解的意思，病邪在表可汗，在里可下，倘在半表半里既不可汗又不可下，病情又正在发展，就需要一种较为和缓的方法来驱除病邪，故和解法用在外感症方面，其主要目的仍在驱邪外出。在杂病方面使用和法，意义稍异。例如血虚劳热，纳食减少，妇女月经不调，可用调和肝脾的方法。又如胸满不痛，嘈杂呕恶，痰热交阻，可用辛开苦降和胃的方法。因此和法的应用相当广泛，包括和解少阳，安内攘外，调理气血，舒畅气机，芳化和中，等等。和的目的虽同，和的方法不一。

Transliteration 13.4

4. Hé-fǎ: hé shì hé-jiě de yì-si, bìng-xié zài biǎo kě hàn, zài lǐ kě xià, tǎng zài bàn-biǎo-bàn-lǐ jì-bù kě hàn yòu-bù kě xià, bìng-qíng yòu zhèng-zài fā-zhǎn, jiù xū-yào yī zhǒng jiào wéi hé-huǎn de fāng-fǎ lái qū-chú bìng-xié, gù hé-jiě-fǎ yòng zài wài-gǎn-zhèng fāng-miàn, qí zhǔ-yào mù-dì réng zài qū xié wài chū.

Zài zá-bìng fāng-miàn shǐ-yòng hé-fǎ, yì-yì shāo yì. Lì-rú xuè-xū láo-rè, nà shí jiǎn-shǎo, fù-nǚ yuè-jīng bù tiáo, kě yòng tiáo-he gān pí de fāng-fǎ. Yòu rú xiōng mǎn bù tòng, cáo-zá ǒu è, tán rè jiāo zǔ, kě yòng xīn kāi kǔ jiàng hé wèi de fāng-fǎ. Yīn-cǐ hé-fǎ de yìng-yòng xiāng-dāng guǎng-fàn, bāo-kuò hé jiě shào-yáng, ān nèi rǎng wài, tiáo-lǐ qì xuè, shū-chàng qì-jī, fāng huà hé zhōng, děng-děng. Hé de mù-dì suī tóng, hé de fāng-fǎ bù-yī.

Vocabulary 13.4

和法	hé-fǎ	the pattern of harmonization
正在	zhèng-zài	be just (in a specific state)
和缓	hé-huǎn	mild
和解法	hé-jiě-fǎ	pattern of reconciliation
驱	qū	chase away
杂病	zá-bìng	miscellaneous illnesses
劳热	láo-rè	exhaustion heat
减少	jiǎn-shǎo	lessen; decrease
月经	yuè-jīng	monthly period; menstruation
调和	tiáo-he	regulate
嘈杂	cáo-zá	noisy
交	jiāo	unite

攘	rǎng	defense; defend
调理	tiáo-lǐ	regulate
芳	fāng	aromatic
芳化	fāng-huà	transform (dampness) by means of fragrant (drugs)
不一	bù-yī	different

Translation 13.4

4. The pattern of harmonization: Harmonization has the meaning of reconciliation. When a pathogenic evil is in the (body's) outside, sweating can be induced; when it is inside, it is possible to purge. However, when it is half outside and half inside, then it is impossible to induce sweating or to purge. Also, if the nature of the illness is just unfolding, a relatively mild approach is required to remove the evil (causing the) illness. Hence when the pattern of reconciliation is used in cases of pathoconditions (resulting from) exogenous affections, its main objective is nevertheless to chase the evil to leave towards the outside.

When the harmonizing pattern is applied against miscellaneous illnesses (other than those caused by an external evil), the rationale is slightly different. For instance, in case of blood depletion with taxation heat, if less and less food is consumed, or when the monthly periods of women are out of order, it is possible to employ a (therapeutic) pattern to regulate liver and spleen. Or, when (the patient experiences a feeling of) fullness in the chest without pain, when (the patient) vomits bad (things) with great noise, when phlegm and heat unite and form blockages, a pattern to open (passages) with acrid (drugs), and to purge with bitter (drugs) can be employed to harmonize the stomach. From this it follows that the application of the pattern of harmonization is comparatively broad; it includes reconciliation of minor yang (illnesses), pacification of the interior with (simultaneous) defense against external (intruders), regulation of qi and blood, relaxation of the qi dynamics, harmonization of the (abdominal) center by means of fragrant (drugs) transforming (dampness), and so on. Even though the objective of these harmonizations is always identical, the approaches to achieve a harmonization differ.

5. 清法：凡用清凉剂来治疗温热病症，都称清法。温热症候有表热，里热，虚热，实热，气分热，血分热，用清凉剂时必须分辨热的性质及在哪一部分。比如表热症应取辛凉，里热中虚症采用甘寒，实症采用苦寒。在气分清气，在血分清血。清法里包括镇静和解毒，例如肝阳或肝火上扰，头晕头胀，用清肝方剂能使熄风镇痛；还有温毒症用清热凉营。临症上用清解法比较多，但亦不宜多用久用，尤其是苦寒一类的药，能损害脾胃，影响消化。体质素虚，脏腑本寒，食欲不强，大便溏薄，以及产后病后，均宜慎用。

Transliteration 13.5

5. Qīng-fǎ: fán yòng qīng-liáng-jì lái zhì-liáo wēn-rè bìng-zhèng, dōu chēng qīng-fǎ. Wēn-rè zhèng-hòu yǒu biǎo-rè, lǐ-rè, xū-rè, shí-rè, qì-fèn-rè, xuè-fèn-rè, yòng qīng-liáng-jì shí bì-xū fēn-biàn rè de xìng-zhì jí zài nǎ-yī bù-fèn. Bǐ-rú biǎo-rè-zhèng yīng qǔ xīn liáng, lǐ-rè zhōng-xū-zhèng cǎi-yòng gān hán, shí-zhèng cǎi-yòng kǔ hán. Zài qì-fèn qīng qì, zài xuè-fèn qīng xuè.

Qīng-fǎ lǐ bāo-kuò zhèn-jìng hé jiě-dú, lì-rú gān-yáng huò gān-huǒ shàng-rǎo, tóu-yūn tóu-zhàng, yòng qīng gān fāng-jì néng shǐ xī fēng zhèn tòng; hái-yǒu wēn-dú-zhèng yòng qīng-rè liáng yíng.

Lín-zhèng shàng yòng qīng-jiě-fǎ bǐ-jiào duō, dàn yì bù-yí duō yòng jiǔ yòng, yóu qí shì kǔ hán yī lèi de yào, néng sǔn-hài pí wèi, yǐng-xiǎng xiāo-huà. Tǐ-zhì sù xū, zàng-fǔ běn hán, shí-yù bù qiáng, dà-biàn táng-bó, yǐ-jí chǎn hòu bìng hòu, jūn yí shèn yòng.

Vocabulary 13.5

清法	qīng-fǎ	the pattern of cooling
表热	biǎo-rè	exterior heat
里热	lǐ-rè	internal heat
虚热	xū-rè	depletion heat
气分热	qì-fèn-rè	heat in the qi section

血分热	xuè-fèn-rè	heat in the blood section
表热(症)	biǎo-rè-(zhèng)	(pathocondition of) exterior heat
里热(症)	lǐ-rè-(zhèng)	(pathocondition of) internal heat
中虚(症)	zhōng-xū-(zhèng)	(pathocondition of) central depletion
采用	cǎi-yòng	select
血分	xuè-fèn	blood section
镇静	zhèn-jìng	tranquilize
解毒	jiě-dú	detoxify
肝阳	gān-yáng	liver yang
上扰	shàng-rǎo	rise to cause harassment above
方剂	fāng-jì	formula
熄	xī	calm down
镇	zhèn	press down
温毒症	wēn-dú-zhèng	pathocondition of warmth poisoning
营	yíng	blood; constructive (qi)
清解法	qīng-jiě-fǎ	pattern of resolution through cooling
尤其是	yóu-qí-shì	especially
素	sù	since birth
慎	shèn	careful

Translation 13.5

5. The pattern of cooling: All applications of cooling remedies to treat pathoconditions of warmth and heat are called pattern of cooling. The symptomatic pathoconditions of warmth and heat include exterior heat, internal heat, depletion heat, repletion heat, heat in the qi section, and heat in the blood section. When using cooling remedies, it is necessary to differentiate the nature and the location of the heat. For example, in case of a pathocondition of exterior heat it is apppropriate to use acrid and

cool (drugs), in case of a pathocondition of internal heat and central depletion, sweet and cold (drugs) are selected for use; in case of a pathocondition of repletion, bitter and cold (drugs) are selected for use. In the qi section (the therapist) cools the qi; in the blood section (the therapist) cools the blood.

The pattern of cooling includes tranquilization and detoxification. For example, when the liver yang or the liver fire rise and cause harassment above (with the effect that) the head turns dizzy or feels full, a formula is used to cool the liver which may calm the wind and suppress the pain. There are, in addition, pathoconditions of warmth poisoning (requiring the) application of (drugs that) cool the heat and (that) cool the blood.

In clinical practice (Chinese medicine) relatively often uses the pattern of achieving relief through cooling. However, (in the treatment of one and the same patient) it must be used neither frequently nor over an extended period of time. Especially drugs of a bitter and cold nature are quite able to harm the spleen and the stomach, and to influence digestion. When the physical constitution is weak since birth, or when the depots and palaces are cold by nature, when there is no strong desire to eat, when the stools are semi-liquid, and after parturition as well as after an illness, it is always advisable to be careful with an application (of the cooling pattern).

6. 温法：常用于寒性病。寒性病有表寒，里寒等区别，但从温法来说，一般都指里寒，故以温中为主要治法。例如呕吐清水，大便溏薄泄泻，腹痛喜按，手足厥冷，脉象沉伏迟微，均为温法的对象。寒性病有寒邪直中内脏引起的，也有因阳虚而逐渐形成的，所以温法的使用，或以逐寒为主，或以扶阳为主。但逐寒的目的为了防止伤阳，也叫回阳，扶阳也为了祛除沉寒痼冷，两者之间是互有关系的。

Transliteration 13.6

6. Wēn-fǎ: cháng-yòng yú hán-xìng-bìng. Hán-xìng-bìng yǒu biǎo-hán, lǐ-hán děng qū-bié, dàn cóng wēn-fǎ lái shuō, yī-bān dōu zhǐ lǐ-hán, gù yǐ wēn-zhōng wéi zhǔ-yào zhì-fǎ. Lì-rú ǒu-tù qīng-shuǐ, dà-biàn táng-bó xiè-xiè, fù-tòng xǐ àn, shǒu zú jué-lěng, mài-xiàng chén fú chí wēi, jūn wéi wēn-fǎ de duì-xiàng.

Hán-xìng-bìng yǒu hán-xié zhí zhòng nèi-zàng yǐn-qǐ de, yě yǒu yīn yáng-xū ér zhú-jiàn xíng-chéng de, suǒ-yǐ wēn-fǎ de shǐ-yòng, huò yǐ zhú-hán wéi zhǔ, huò yǐ fú-yáng wéi zhǔ. Dàn zhú-hán de mù-dì wéi-le fáng-zhǐ shāng yáng, yě jiào huí-yáng, fú-yáng yě wéi-le qū-chú chén-hán gù-lěng, liǎng zhě zhī-jiān shì hù yǒu guān-xi de.

Vocabulary 13.6

寒性病	hán-xìng-bìng	illnesses of a cold nature
对象	duì-xiàng	target
逐渐	zhú-jiàn	slowly; gradually
逐寒	zhú-hán	eliminate cold
扶阳	fú-yáng	support the yang
祛除	qū-chú	eliminate
沉寒	chén-hán	deep-seated cold
互	hù	mutual

Translation 13.6

6. The pattern of warming: It is regularly applied in the treatment of illnesses of a cold nature. Among the illnesses of a cold nature, a difference exists, among others, between outside cold and inside cold. In general, though, the pattern of warming is directed at (a treatment of) inside cold. Hence its major therapeutic approach is to warm the (body's) center. For instance, when someone vomits clear water, when the stools

are semi-liquid or in case of diarrhea, in case of abdominal pain with pressure (exerted there causing) comfort, when hands and feet turn cold because of recession (of yang qi), and when the pulse appears deep and hidden, retarded and feeble, then all these (conditions) are targets of the warming pattern.

Illnesses of a cold nature may emerge because cold evil strikes the depots in the interior directly, or they slowly take form as a consequence of a yang depletion. Hence an application of the warming pattern has as its main objective either the elimination of the cold, or the support of the yang. However, the objective of eliminating the cold is to prevent the yang from harm, it is also called "making the yang return," and the support of the yang, in turn, aims at eliminating deep-seated cold and obstinate frigidity. Between these two (approaches) there exist mutual relationships.

7. 消法：主要是消导，用来消除肠胃壅滞，例如食积内阻，脘服胀满，治以消化导下。其次是消坚，多用于凝结成形的病症，如癥瘕积聚和瘰疬等，因为这类病症多由气血停滞，其来也渐，其去也亦缓，不是攻逐所能荡尽，须用磨运消散，缓以图功。再次是消痰，痰浊的原因不一，有寒痰，湿痰，痰热以及顽痰等，故须分别用温化，清化，涤痰，豁痰等方法，总称消痰。还有利水亦在消法之内。水湿以走小便为顺，如果水湿内停，小便不利，或走大便而成泄泻，应予利导，使之从小便排出，一般称为利尿，亦叫淡渗。

Transliteration 13.7

7. Xiāo-fǎ: zhǔ-yào shì xiāo dǎo, yòng lái xiāo-chú cháng wèi yōng-zhì, lì-rú shí-jī nèi-zǔ, wǎn fù zhàng-mǎn, zhì yǐ xiāo-huà dǎo-xià. Qí-cì shì xiāo jiān, duō yòng yú níng-jié chéng-xíng de bìng-zhèng, rú zhēng-jiǎ jī-jù hé luǒ-lì děng, yīn-wéi zhè-lèi bìng-zhèng duō yóu qì xuè tíng-zhì, qí lái yě jiàn, qí qù yě yì huǎn, bù shì gōng zhú suǒ néng dàng jìn, xū yòng mó yùn xiāo sàn, huǎn yǐ tú gōng. Zài-cì shì xiāo tán, tán-zhuó de yuán-yīn bù-yī, yǒu hán-tán, shī-tán, tán-rè yǐ-jí wán-tán děng, gù xū fēn-bié yòng wēn-huà, qīng-huà, dí-tán, huō-tán děng fāng-fǎ, zǒng chēng xiāo-tán.

Hái-yǒu lì-shuǐ yì zài xiāo-fǎ zhī nèi. Shuǐ-shī yǐ zǒu xiǎo-biàn wéi shùn, rú-guǒ shuǐ-shī nèi tíng, xiǎo-biàn bù lì, huò zǒu dà-biàn ér chéng xiè-xiè, yīng yǔ lì-dǎo, shǐ zhī cóng xiǎo-biàn pái chū, yī-bān chēng-wéi lì-niào, yì jiào dàn-shèn.

Vocabulary 13.7

消法	xiāo-fǎ	the pattern of dissolving
导	dǎo	guide
消除	xiāo-chú	eliminate
壅滞	yōng-zhì	obstruction
内阻	nèi-zǔ	internal blockage
导下	dǎo-xià	guide downwards
凝结	níng-jié	coagulate

成形	chéng-xíng	assume physical shape
癥瘕	zhèng-jiǎ	concretion
积聚	jī-jù	conglomeration
渐	jiàn	gradually
荡	dàng	sweep away
尽	jìn	completely
磨	mó	grind
图	tú	plan
功	gōng	success
再次	zài-cì	still another
痰热	tán-rè	phlegm heat
顽痰	wán-tán	obstinate phlegm
温化	wēn-huà	transformation by means of warmth
清化	qīng-huà	transformation by means of cooling
涤痰	dí-tán	flush away phlegm
豁痰	huō-tán	clear away phlegm
消痰	xiāo-tán	dissolve phlegm
利水	lì-shuǐ	diuresis
顺	shùn	appropriate
停	tíng	stagnate
利导	lì-dǎo	free (a passage) and guide (there)
排	pái	emit
利尿	lì-niào	free urination
淡渗	dàn-shèn	bland seeping

Translation 13.7

7. The pattern of dissolving: (This approach) consists mainly of dissolving and guiding; it is employed to eliminate obstructions in the intestines and in the stomach. For example, internal blockages resulting from food accumulations, and distensions and fullness in the (gastric) cavity and in

the abdomen, are treated through dissolving transformation and guiding downwards. The second (approach) consists in dissolving solid (items); it is often used against illnesses where coagulations have assumed physical shape, such as accumulations of concretions and conglomerations and scrofulous lumps, because such pathoconditions often result from a stagnation of qi or blood. They emerge gradually, and they also vanish slowly. They cannot be swept away completely through an attack; they must be dissolved and dispersed with a grinding movement. Success should be sought without hurry. Another (approach) is to transform phlegm. The causes of phlegm turbidity vary; there are cold phlegm; damp phlegm, phlegm heat, and also obstinate phlegm. Hence it is necessary to distinguish among an application of patterns such as transformation by means of warmth, transformation by means of cooling, phlegm flushing[1], and phlegm clearing.[2] Together (these approaches) are called dissolving phlegm.

The pattern of dissolving includes also diuresis. Water dampness should leave (the body with the) urine. When dampness stagnates inside (the body), and when the urine does not flow freely, or when (the dampness) goes the way of the stools and produces diarrhea, it is advisable to free (its usual path) and guide (it there) so that it is emitted together with the urine. This is generally called freeing urination; it is also called "bland seeping."

Notes

1 A therapy pattern employing drugs dissolving, that is, "flushing" the phlegm.

2 A therapy pattern employing drugs stimulating a forceful throw up of phlegm through coughing.

8. 补法：就是补充体力不足，从而消除一切衰弱症候，故内经说："虚者补之"。所用药物大多含有滋养性质，故亦称滋补，补养。补法在临症上分补气，补血，益精，安神，生津液，填骨髓等，总之，以强壮为目的。补剂的性质可分三种，一为温补，用于阳虚症；一为清补，用于阴虚症；另一种为平补，用于一般虚弱症。由于病情的轻重不同，又分为峻补和缓补。峻补常用于积弱极虚之体，或以急救为目的换回虚脱；缓补则用于体质虽虚不胜重补，或虚而别无大寒大热症状，只宜和平之剂缓缓调养。

Transliteration 13.8

8. Bǔ-fǎ: jiù-shì bǔ-chōng tǐ-lì bù-zú, cóng-ér xiāo-chú yī-qiè shuāi-ruò zhèng-hòu, gù nèi-jīng shuō: "Xū zhě bǔ zhī." Suǒ yòng yào-wù dà-duō hán-yǒu zī-yǎng xìng-zhì, gù yì chēng zī-bǔ, bǔ-yǎng.

Bǔ-fǎ zài lín-zhèng shàng fēn bǔ-qì, bǔ-xuè, yì-jīng, ān-shén, shēng-jīn-yè, tián-gǔ-suí děng, zǒng-zhī, yǐ qiáng-zhuàng wéi mù-dì.

Bǔ-jì de xìng-zhì kě fēn sān zhǒng, yī wéi wēn-bǔ, yòng yú yáng-xū-zhèng; yī wéi qīng-bǔ, yòng yú yīn-xū-zhèng; lìng-yī zhǒng wéi píng-bǔ, yòng yú yī-bān xū ruò zhèng.

Yóu-yú bìng-qíng de qīng zhòng bù-tóng, yòu fēn-wéi jùn-bǔ hé huǎn-bǔ. Jùn-bǔ cháng-yòng yú jī-ruò jí-xū zhī tǐ, huò yǐ jí jiù wéi mù-dì wǎn-huí xū-tuō; huǎn-bǔ zé yòng yú tǐ-zhì suī xū bù shèng zhòng bǔ, huò xū ér bié wú dà hán dà rè zhèng-zhuàng, zhǐ yí hé-píng zhī jì huǎn-huǎn tiáo-yǎng.

Vocabulary 13.8

补充	bǔ-chōng	supplement
补养	bǔ-yǎng	tonify
补血	bǔ-xuè	supplement the blood
益精	yì-jīng	increase the semen
生津液	shēng-jīn-yè	generate body liquids

填骨髓	tián-gǔ-suí	fill the bone marrow
总之	zǒng-zhī	in general; to sum up
强壮	qiáng-zhuàng	strengthen; be strong
温补	wēn-bǔ	warm supplementation
阳虚症	yáng-xū-zhèng	pathocondition of yang depletion
清补	qīng-bǔ	cool supplementation
阴虚症	yīn-xū-zhèng	pathocondition of yin depletion
平补	píng-bǔ	balanced supplementation
峻补	jùn-bǔ	drastic supplementation
缓补	huǎn-bǔ	mild supplementation
积弱	jī-ruò	very weak
极虚	jí-xū	extreme depletion
挽回	wǎn-huí	retrieve
虚脱	xū-tuō	loss
别	bié	additional
和平	hé-píng	balanced
缓缓	huǎn-huǎn	mildly

Translation 13.8

8. The pattern of supplementation: (This pattern) serves to supplement any insufficiencies in the body's strength, and thereby to eliminate all pathoconditions of weakness. Hence the *Neijing* states: "If it is depleted, supplement it." Most of the drugs applied here have a nourishing nature; hence (Chinese medicine) also speaks of "nourishing supplementation" and "supplementing tonification."

The pattern of supplementation is divided, in clinical practice, into (approaches aiming at) supplementing the qi, supplementing the blood, increasing the semen, calming the spirit, generating body liquids, and filling the bone marrow. In general, the objective is a strengthening.

The nature of supplementing remedies can be divided into three types. One causes warm supplementation; it is used against pathoconditions of yang depletion. One causes cool supplementation; it is used against pathoconditions of yin depletion. Another type causes balanced supplementation; it is used against pathoconditions of general weakness.

Because the severity of the illnesses may differ, (Chinese medicine) distinguishes, in addition, between drastic supplementation and mild supplementation. Drastic supplementation is used regularly on bodies that are very weak or extremely depleted, or to provide emergency help in retrieving a loss. Mild supplementation, then, is used in cases where the physical constitution may be weak but would not stand heavy supplementation; or where a depletion exists without additional pathoconditions of strong cold or strong heat. Here it is appropriate to regulate mildly with remedies of a balanced (nature).

Text 14.1

用多种药物配成的处方，称做方剂。方剂的组成有一定的法度，称做方制。所以，方剂是用单味药物治疗的进一步发展。它的特点是：具有综合作用，治疗范围较广，并能调和药物的毒性，减少或避免不良反应。方剂的组成，分君，臣，佐，使四项。一般处方用药多在四种以上，均按这四项配伍，即使少于四种药或多至几十种，也不能离此法则。否则漫无纪律，方向不明，前人所谓有药无方。

Transliteration 14.1

Yòng duō zhǒng yào-wù pèi-chéng de chǔ-fāng, chēng-zuò fāng-jì. Fāng-jì de zǔ-chéng yǒu yī-dìng de fǎ-dù, chēng-zuò fāng-zhì. Suǒ-yǐ, fāng-jì shì yòng dān-wèi yào-wù zhì-liáo de jìn-yī-bù fā-zhǎn. Tā-de tè-diǎn shì: jù-yǒu zōng-hé zuò-yòng, zhì-liáo fàn-wéi jiào guǎng, bìng néng tiáo-he yào-wù de dú-xìng, jiǎn-shǎo huò bì-miǎn bù-liáng fǎn-yìng.

Fāng-jì de zǔ-chéng, fēn jūn, chén, zuǒ, shǐ sì-xiàng. Yī-bān chǔ-fāng yòng yào duō zài sì zhǒng yǐ-shàng, jūn àn zhè sì-xiàng pèi-wǔ, jí shǐ shǎo yú sì zhǒng yào huò duō zhì jǐ-shí zhǒng, yě bù néng lí cǐ fǎ-zé. Fǒu zé màn-wú jì-lǜ, fāng-xiàng bù míng, qián-rén suǒ-wèi yǒu yào wú fāng.

Vocabulary 14.1

配成	pèi-chéng	combine
法度	fǎ-dù	law
方制	fāng-zhì	system of prescribing
味	wèi	(measure word for drugs)
单味	dān-wèi	single drugs
综合	zōng-hé	comprehensive
毒性	dú-xìng	toxicity
避免	bì-miǎn	avoid
反应	fǎn-yìng	reaction
君	jūn	ruler
臣	chén	minister
使	shǐ	messenger
四项	sì-xiàng	the four components (in structuring a prescription)
配伍	pèi-wǔ	compose
使	shǐ	if; given
几十	jǐ-shí	tens of
离	lí	leave; defy; go against

漫无	màn-wú	there is/are absolutely no ...
纪律	jì-lǜ	discipline

Translation 14.1

Formulas made up by a combination of numerous kinds of drugs are called prescriptions. The structure of prescriptions follows a firm law; it is called system of prescribing. That is to say, prescriptions are a further development of the application of single drugs for therapy. Their characteristics are: they have a comprehensive action; their therapeutic range is comparatively broad; and they enable (a therapist) to regulate the toxicity of drug-substances, and to decrease or avoid unwanted reactions.

In the structure of prescriptions (Chinese medicine) distinguishes the four components of ruler, minister, assistant, and messenger. In general, more than four kinds of drugs are applied in a formula, and all of them are composed in accordance with (the hierarchy among) these four components. Even if (a prescription combines) less than four drugs, or as many as tens (of drugs), this rule must not be defied nevertheless. Otherwise there will be absolutely no discipline, the direction (of the treatment) will be unclear, and this is what the people in former times called "drugs are present, but there is no formula."

1. 君：君是一方的主药，针对一病的主因，主症能起主要作用的药物。君药不一定一方只有一个，也不一定猛烈的药才能当君药，主要是看具体情况和需要来决定的。

2. 臣：内经上说："佐君之谓臣"。臣是指协助和加强君药效能的药物，如麻黄汤中的桂枝就是帮助麻黄发汗解表的，所以它在麻黄汤中是臣药。臣药在一个方剂内，不限定只有一味。如果一方中有两个君药，还能用较多的臣药来配伍。

Transliteration 14.2

1. Jūn: jūn shì yī fāng de zhǔ-yào, zhēn-duì yī bìng de zhǔ-yīn, zhǔ-zhèng néng qǐ zhǔ-yào zuò-yòng de yào-wù. Jūn-yào bù-yī-dìng yī fāng zhǐ yǒu yī ge, yě bù-yī-dìng měng-liè de yào cái néng dāng jūn-yào, zhǔ-yào shì kàn jù-tǐ qíng-kuàng hé xū-yào lái jué-dìng de.

2. Chén: nèi-jīng shàng shuō: "zuǒ jūn zhī wèi chén." Chén shì zhǐ xié-zhù hé jiā-qiáng jūn-yào xiào-néng de yào-wù, rú má-huáng-tāng zhōng de guì-zhī jiù-shì bāng-zhù má-huáng fā-hàn jiě biǎo de, suǒ-yǐ tā zài má-huáng-tāng zhōng shì chén-yào. Chén-yào zài yī ge fāng-jì nèi, bù xiàn-dìng zhǐ yǒu yī wèi. Rú-guǒ yī fāng zhōng yǒu liǎng gè jūn-yào, hái néng yòng jiào duō de chén-yào lái pèi-wǔ.

Vocabulary 14.2

君药	jūn-yào	ruler drug
不一定	bù-yī-dìng	not necessarily
看 ... 来 ...	kàn ... lái ...	observe ... to ...; (do something) on the basis of ...
协助	xié-zhù	support
效能	xiào-néng	effect
麻黄汤	má-huáng-tāng	decoction with mahuang
桂枝	guì-zhī	(drug name) Cinnamomum cassia Blume
臣药	chén-yào	minister drug
限定	xiàn-dìng	restricted

Translation 14.2

1. The ruler: The ruler is the main drug in a formula. It is the drug which is able to exert the major effect against the main cause and against the main pathoconditions of an illness. It is not necessarily such that one

single formula has only one ruler drug; and it is not necessarily a violent drug that may serve as a ruler drug. It is important to decide on the basis of the actual situation and requirements (which drug is to be employed as ruler drug).

2. The ministers: The *Neijing* states: “He who assists the ruler is called minister.” The (term) minister refers to drugs that support and strengthen the effects of the ruler drug. For example, in the “decoction with mahuang” guizhi helps the mahuang to induce sweating and open the outside. Hence it serves as minister drug in the decoction with mahuang. Minister drugs are not restricted to only one substance per prescription. If there are two ruler drugs within one formula, it is advisable to apply, in addition, a relatively large number of minister drugs to accompany them.

3. 佐：臣之下称做佐，佐药就是接近于臣药的一种配伍药。除了与臣药一样协助君药的作用，还能协助君药解除某些次要症状。例如麻黄汤用杏仁为佐，其作用就是宣肺，平喘，帮助君药解除麻黄汤症的次要症状。另一方面，假使君药有毒性或者药性太偏，也可利用佐药来调和。

4. 使：从使字的意义来看，使药是一方内比较最次要的药物。内经说："应臣之为使"。可知使药是臣药的一种辅助药。在临症上一般把使药理解为引经药，引经药的意思是将药力引到发病场所，所以也叫引药。

Transliteration 14.3

3. Zuǒ: chén zhī xià chēng-zuò zuǒ, zuǒ-yào jiù-shì jiē-jìn yú chén-yào de yī zhǒng pèi-wǔ yào. Chú-le yǔ chén-yào yī-yàng xié-zhù jūn-yào de zuò-yòng, hái néng xié-zhù jūn-yào jiě-chú mǒu-xiē cì-yào zhèng-zhuàng. Lì-rú má-huáng-tāng yòng xìng-rén wéi zuǒ, qí zuò-yòng jiù-shì xuān fèi, píng chuǎn, bāng-zhù jūn-yào jiě-chú má-huáng-tāng zhèng de cì-yào zhèng-zhuàng. Lìng-yī fāng-miàn, jiǎ-shǐ jūn-yào yǒu dú-xìng huòzhe yào-xìng tài piān, yě kě lì-yòng zuǒ-yào lái tiáo-he.

4. Shǐ: cóng shǐ zì de yì-yì lái kàn, shǐ-yào shì yī fāng nèi bǐ-jiào zuì cì-yào de yào-wù. Nèi-jīng shuō: "yīng chén zhī wéi shǐ." Kě-zhī shǐ-yào shì chén-yào de yī zhǒng fǔ-zhù-yào. Zài lín-zhèng shàng yī-bān bǎ shǐ-yào lǐ-jiě wéi yǐn-jīng-yào, yǐn-jīng-yào de yì-si shì jiāng yào-lì yǐn-dào fā-bìng chǎng-suǒ, suǒ-yǐ yě jiào yǐn-yào.

Vocabulary 14.3

佐药	zuǒ-yào	assistant drug
接近	jiē-jìn	be close to (someone/something)
杏仁	xìng-rén	(drug name) Prunus armeniaca L.
宣	xuān	disperse
喘	chuǎn	pant
或者	huò-zhě	or if

太	tài	too much
利用	lì-yòng	use; make use of
使药	shǐ-yào	messenger drug
可知	kě-zhī	it can be realized
辅助药	fǔ-zhù-yào	helper drug
引经药	yǐn-jīng-yào	conduit guiding drug
药力	yào-lì	drug force
引到	yǐn-dào	guide
场所	chǎng-suǒ	location
引药	yǐn-yào	guiding drug

Translation 14.3

3. The assistants: (The position) below the minister is called "assistant." Assistant drugs are a kind of accompanying drugs close to the minister drugs. In addition to their supporting the effects of the ruler drugs in the same way as the minister drugs, they can also help the ruler drugs in the elimination of certain secondary pathoconditions. For example, in the "decoction with mahuang," xingren is used as an assistant; its function is to disperse lung (qi), to calm the panting, and to help the ruler drug to eliminate the secondary pathoconditions among those pathoconditions (against which) the "decoction with mahuang" (is directed). Furthermore, if the ruler drug has a toxic nature, or if the nature of the (ruler) drug is too onesided, it is also possible to make use of assistant drugs to achieve a balance.

4. The messengers: Seen from the meaning of the term "messenger," the messenger drugs constitute – in comparison – the most subordinate substances in a drug formula. The *Neijing* states: "Those who respond to the minister's (beck and call), they are the messengers." (From this any student) can realize that the messenger drugs are a kind of helper drugs to the minister drugs. In clinical practice, the messenger drugs are generally perceived as conduit guiding drugs. The meaning of conduit guiding drugs is that they guide the force of (other) drugs to the location where an illness has emerged. Hence they are called "guiding drugs."

中医从单味药的使用发展到方剂，这是很早以前的事。到张仲景博采众方撰述"伤寒论"和"金匮要略"，方剂更为完备。后人重视其著作尊为经典，并称其方为经方，把后来方剂叫做时方。我们认为经方的疗效是肯定了的，但时方的价值也是不可否认的。时方的形成，也是中医学术不断发展的例证之一。同样的理由，上面说过的六经辨症法是以"伤寒论"为主，三焦辨症法是以"温病条辨"为主，一在汉朝，一在清代，不仅没有抵触，而且相得益彰。"温病条辨"的方剂在"伤寒论"的基础上还有不少的发挥和补充。所以，在古为今用的目标下，我们应重视经方，也应重视时方，还要重视现代的有效方剂。

Transliteration 14.4

Zhōng-yī cóng dān-wèi-yào de shǐ-yòng fā-zhǎn dào fāng-jì, zhè shì hěn zǎo yǐ-qián de shì. Dào zhāng zhòng-jǐng bó cǎi zhòng fāng zhuàn-shù “shāng-hán-lùn” hé “jīn-guì-yào-lüè,” fāng-jì gèng wéi wán-bèi. Hòu-rén zhòng-shì qí zhù-zuò zūn-wéi jīng-diǎn, bìng chēng qí fāng wéi jīng-fāng, bǎ hòu-lái fāng-jì jiào-zuò shí-fāng. Wǒ-men rèn-wéi jīng-fāng de liáo-xiào shì kěn-dìng le de, dàn shí-fāng de jià-zhí yě shì bù-kě fǒu-rèn de. Shí-fāng de xíng-chéng, yě shì zhōng-yī xué-shù bù-duàn fā-zhǎn de lì-zhèng zhī yī. Tóng-yàng de lǐ-yóu, shàng-miàn shuō guò de liù-jīng biàn-zhèng-fǎ shì yǐ “shāng-hán-lùn” wéi zhǔ, sān-jiāo biàn-zhèng-fǎ shì yǐ “wēn-bìng-tiáo-biàn” wéi zhǔ, yī zài hàn-cháo, yī zài qīng-dài, bù-jǐn méi yǒu dǐ-chù, ér-qiě xiāng dé yì zhāng. “Wēn-bìng-tiáo-biàn” de fāng-jì zài “shāng-hán-lùn” de jī-chǔ shàng hái-yǒu bù shǎo de fā-huī hé bǔ-chōng. Suǒ-yǐ, zài gǔ wéi jīn yòng de mù-biāo xià, wǒ-men yīng zhòng-shì jīng-fāng, yě yīng zhòng-shì shí-fāng, hái yào zhòng-shì xiàn-dài de yǒu-xiào fāng-jì.

Vocabulary 14.4

单味药	dān-wèi-yào	single substance drug
早	zǎo	early
以前	yǐ-qián	before; in the past
张仲景	zhāng zhòng-jǐng	(author's name) Zhang Zhong-jing
博	bó	in large measure; comprehensively
采	cǎi	collect
众	zhòng	numerous
撰述	zhuàn-shù	compile
金匮要略	jīn-guì-yào-lüè	(book title:) "Important (Prescriptions) from the Golden Chest"
完备	wán-bèi	perfect; complete
著作	zhù-zuò	writing
尊为	zūn-wéi	revere as
经典	jīng-diǎn	classic
经方	jīng-fāng	classic formulas
后来	hòu-lái	later one
时方	shí-fāng	formulas (introduced in later) times
疗效	liáo-xiào	therapeutic efficacy
肯定	kěn-dìng	confirm
否认	fǒu-rèn	deny
学术	xué-shù	science
不断	bù-duàn	continuous
例证	lì-zhèng	example
上面	shàng-miàn	above
过	guò	(particle indicating the conclusion of the process expressed by the immediately preceding verb)

辨症法	biàn-zhèng-fǎ	pattern to distinguish between pathoconditions
温病条辨	wēn-bìng-tiáo-biàn	(book title:) "Heat Illnesses Discussed in Individual Paragraphs"
汉朝	hàn-cháo	the Han dynasty (206 BCE to 221 CE)
清代	qīng-dài	the Qing dynasty (1644-1912)
不仅 ... 而且 ...	bù-jǐn ... ér-qiě ...	not only ... also ...
抵触	dǐ-chù	be in conflict
相得益彰	xiāng dé yì zhāng	be of mutual complementarity
发挥	fā-huī	elaborate
今	jīn	now; today
古为今用	gǔ wéi jīn yòng	make the old useful for today
目标	mù-biāo	objective
现代	xiàn-dài	present

Translation 14.4

The development in Chinese medicine from an application of single substance drugs to prescriptions is something that has happened a long time ago. By the time Zhang Zhongjing had collected numerous formulas and compiled the *Shanghan lun* as well as the *Jingui yaolüe*,[1] (the art of formulating) prescriptions had been perfected. Later people thought highly of these writings, and revered them as "classic codes." Also, they called their formulas "classic formulas," and they designated the formulas (introduced) later on as "formulas (introduced in later) times." In our opinion, the therapeutic efficacy of the classic formulas has been confirmed, but the value of the formulas (introduced in later) times should not be denied either. The formation of the formulas (that were introduced in later) times is another example of a continuous development of Chinese medical science. For the same reason, there is not only no conflict, but mutual complementarity, when the above-mentioned pattern of distinguishing among the pathoconditions by (investigating) the six conduits is based on the *Shanghan lun*, and when the pattern of distinguishing the pathoconditions by (investigating) the triple burner is based on the *Wenbing tiaobian, the* former being (a work) of the Han dynasty, the latter being (a work) of the Qing dynasty. The prescriptions of the *Wenbing tiaobian* contain many elaborations and supplementations on the basis of the *Shanghan lun*. Hence, under the objective of making the old useful for today, we should think highly of the classic formulas, and we should also think highly of the formulas (introduced in later) times, and, furthermore, we should think highly of effective formulas of the present.

Notes

1 On Zhang Zhongjing (i.e., Zhang Ji) see Text 9.1, Note 2.

2 The *Wenbing tiaobian* was compiled in 1798 by Wu Tang 吴瑭 .

Text 14.5

方剂在应用上，由于所用药物的种类多少和产生疗效的快慢不同，又分为七类，简称七方，即大方，小方，缓方，急方，奇方，偶方和复方。

1. 大方：病邪强盛，非大力不能克制，须用大方，如下法中的大承气汤便是。用大方的时候，应先考虑正气能否胜任，因为大下可以伤阴，大汗可使亡阳，邪虽去而正气随伤，这就失却用大方的意义了。

2. 小方：小方和大方是相对的。邪气轻浅的，只要用较轻的方剂，或者根据大方减小其制，这就叫做小方，如下法中的小承气汤便是。

3.缓方：一般慢性，虚弱性病症，不能急切求效，宜用药力缓和的方剂来长期调养。

Transliteration 14.5

Fāng-jì zài yìng-yòng shàng, yóu-yú suǒ yòng yào-wù de zhǒng-lèi duō-shǎo hé chǎn-shēng liáo-xiào de kuài-màn bù-tóng, yòu fēn-wéi qī lèi, jiǎn chēng qī-fāng, jí dà-fāng, xiǎo-fāng, huǎn-fāng, jí-fāng, jī-fāng, ǒu-fāng hé fù-fāng.

1. Dà-fāng: bìng-xié qiáng-shèng, fēi dà lì bù néng kè-zhì, xū yòng dà-fāng, rú xià-fǎ zhōng de dà-chéng-qì-tāng biàn-shì. Yòng dà-fāng de shí-hòu, yīng xiān kǎo-lǜ zhèng-qì néng fǒu shèng-rèn, yīn-wèi dà-xià kě-yǐ shāng yīn, dà-hàn kě shǐ wáng yáng, xié suī qù ér zhèng-qì suí shāng, zhè jiù shī-què yòng dà-fāng de yì-yì le.

2. Xiǎo-fāng: xiǎo-fāng hé dà-fāng shì xiāng-duì de. Xié-qì qīng qiǎn de, zhǐ yào yòng jiào qīng de fāng-jì, huò-zhě gēn-jù dà-fāng jiǎn-xiǎo qí zhì, zhè jiù jiào-zuò xiǎo-fāng, rú xià-fǎ zhōng de xiǎo-chéng-qì-tāng biàn shì.

3. Huǎn-fāng: yī-bān màn-xìng, xū-ruò xìng bìng-zhèng, bù néng jí-qiè qiú xiào, yí yòng yào-lì huǎn-hé de fāng-jì lái cháng-qī tiáo-yǎng.

Vocabulary 14.5

种类	zhǒng-lèi	kind; type
多少	duō-shǎo	many and few; amount
快慢	kuài-màn	fast and slow; speed
七方	qī-fāng	the seven formulas
大方	dà-fāng	large formula
小方	xiǎo-fāng	small formula
缓方	huǎn-fāng	mild formula
急方	jí-fāng	urgent formula
奇方	jī-fāng	unpaired formula
偶方	ǒu-fāng	paired formula
复方	fù-fāng	compound formula
力	lì	strength
便是	biàn-shì	(final particle emphasizing the preceding statement)
如 ... 便是	rú ... biàn-shì	as for example
克制	kè-zhì	overcome
大承气汤	dà-chéng-qì-tāng	large formula to contain the qi
胜任	shèng-rèn	stand (something)
大下	dà-xià	major purgation
大汗	dà-hàn	major sweating
失	shī	miss
失却	shī-què	miss entirely
减小	jiǎn-xiǎo	decrease
制	zhì	scope
小承气汤	xiǎo-chéng-qì-tāng	small decoction to contain the qi
急切	jí-qiè	fast
效	xiào	effect

Translation 14.5

Starting from the differences in the number of the kinds of drugs used, and in the speed with which they produce their therapeutic effects, seven types of prescriptions are distinguished in view of their application. They are called simply the seven formulas, and they include the large formula, the small formula, the mild formula, the urgent formula, the unpaired formula, the paired formula, as well as the compound formula.

1. The large formula: When the pathogenic evil is strong and abounds, and when it can be overcome only by a large force, it is necessary to employ a large formula, as for instance the "large formula to contain the qi" (that is used) in the context of the purgation pattern. When applying a large formula, (a therapist) should first take into consideration whether or not the (patient's) proper qi will be able to stand (such an approach), because a major purgation can harm the yin (qi), and a major sweating can cause a loss of yang (qi). If the evil was eliminated with the proper qi being harmed as a consequence, that would be to miss entirely the meaning of an application of a large formula.

2. The small formula: The small formula and the large formula are opposites. When the evil qi is light and superficial, all that is required is to use merely a comparatively light prescription, or to start from a large formula and decrease its scope. This then is called a small formula. An example is the "small decoction to contain the qi" (that is used) in the context of the purgation pattern.

3. The mild formula: In general, against chronic pathoconditions, or those of a depletion or weakness type, it is impossible to seek fast effects. It is advisable to use prescriptions with drugs whose strength is mild and harmonizing to build up the (patient's) health over an extended period of time.

4. 急方：急方和缓方是相对的。是在病势危急时用来急救的，例如腹泻不止，手足逆冷，脉微欲绝，用四逆汤回阳。急症用急方，不仅药力要专，药量也宜重，故常与大方结合应用。

5. 奇方：奇是单数，奇方即专一的意思。如病因只有一个，就用一种君药来治疗主症，以求其药力专一，故叫奇方。但奇方并不等于单味药，亦有臣药，佐药等配合。

6. 偶方：偶是双数，含有双方兼顾的意思。如同时有两个病因，需要用两种君药来治疗的，就叫偶方。临症上所说的汗下兼施，或攻补并用，都属偶方一类。

Transliteration 14.6

4. Jí-fāng: jí-fāng hé huǎn-fāng shì xiāng-duì de. Shì zài bìng-shì wēi-jí shí yòng lái jí jiù de, lì-rú fù-xiè bù-zhǐ, shǒu zú nì lěng, mài wēi yù jué, yòng sì-nì-tāng huí-yáng. Jí-zhèng yòng jí-fāng, bù-jǐn yào-lì yào zhuān, yào-liàng yě yí zhòng, gù cháng yǔ dà-fāng jié-hé yìng-yòng.

5. Jī-fāng: jī shì dān-shù, jī-fāng jí zhuān-yī de yì-si. Rú bìng-yīn zhǐ-yǒu yī ge, jiù yòng yī zhǒng jūn-yào lái zhì-liáo zhǔ-zhèng, yǐ qiú qí yào-lì zhuān-yī, gù jiào jí-fāng. Dàn jī-fāng bìng bù-děng yú dān-wèi-yào, yì yǒu chén-yào, zuǒ-yào děng pèi-hé.

6. Ōu-fāng: ǒu shì shuāng-shù, hán-yǒu shuāng fāng jiān-gù de yì-si. Rú tóng-shí yǒu liǎng ge bìng-yīn, xū-yào yòng liǎng zhǒng jūn-yào lái zhì-liáo de, jiù jiào ǒu-fāng. Lín-zhèng shàng suǒ-shuō-de hàn xià jiān-shī, huò gōng bǔ bìng-yòng, dōu shǔ ǒu-fāng yī lèi.

Vocabulary 14.6

腹泻	fù-xiè	diarrhea
逆	nì	countermovement; (in medical texts often used as an abbreviation for “qi flowing

		contrary to its normal direction")
四逆汤	sì-nì-tāng	decoction against countermovement (of qi in the) four (limbs)
药量	yào-liàng	quantity of drugs
单数	dān-shù	odd numbers
专一	zhuān-yī	concentrated
不等	bù-děng	not identical
偶	ǒu	paired; even
双数	shuāng-shù	even numbers
双	shuāng	both
并用	bìng-yòng	apply simultaneously; simultaneous application

Translation 14.6

4. The urgent formula: The urgent formula and the mild formula are opposites. (The former) is applied to bring emergency help when the force of an illness has reached a critical stage. For example, in case of incessant diarrhea, when hands and feet turn cold because of a countermovement (of yang qi), when the pulse is feeble and tends to be interrupted entirely, the "decoction against countermovement (of qi in the) four (limbs)" is used to have the yang (qi) return. When urgent formulas are applied against acute pathoconditions, not only the strength of the drugs must be focussed (on the particular problem at hand), the quantities of the drugs must be increased too. Hence (urgent formulas) are often used in combination with large formulas.

5. The unpaired formula: "Unpaired" stands for odd numbers. Hence (the term) unpaired formula carries the meaning of concentrated (formula). For example, if an illness has only one cause, (a therapist) employs just one ruler drug to treat the main pathocondition, thereby taking advantage of the concentrated strength of this particular drug. Hence (such formulas)

are called unpaired formulas. However, unpaired formulas are not identical with single substance drugs; they may also be combinations of (ruler drugs) with minister drugs and assistant drugs.

6. The paired formula: "Paired" stands for even numbers; (the term) carries the meaning of "paying attention to both sides." For instance, if two causes of illness exist simultaneously, it is necessary to use two ruler drugs for their treatment. This is called a paired formula. The so-called simultaneous application of (induced) sweating and purgation, or the concurrent use of attacking and supplementing (drugs) in clinical practice, all (these approaches) belong to the category of "paired formulas."

Text 14.7

7. 复方：复是复杂，重复的意思。凡是病因较多或病情较复杂的就需用复方治疗，如五积散是由麻黄汤，桂枝汤，平胃散和二陈汤等方剂组成，用一方来祛除风，寒，痰，湿以及消痞去积。

七方是方剂组成的法则之一。除此以外，还有从治疗作用来分的。如张景岳曾把方剂分为"八阵"，即补阵，和阵，攻阵，散阵，寒阵，热阵，固阵，因阵。补阵的方剂是用于元气亏损，体质虚弱的病症；和阵的方剂是用来调和病邪的偏胜；攻阵的方剂是用于内实症的；散阵的方剂是用于外感症的；寒阵的方剂是用于热症的；热阵的方剂是用于寒症的；固阵的方剂是用于滑泄不禁症的；因阵的方剂都是因症立方的。

Transliteration 14.7

1. Fù-fāng: fù shì fù-zá, chóng-fù de yì-si. Fán-shì bìng-yīn jiào duō huò bìng-qíng jiào fù-zá de jiù xū yòng fù-fāng zhì-liáo, rú wǔ-jī-sǎn shì yóu má-huáng-tāng, guì-zhī-tāng, píng-wèi-sǎn hé èr-chén-tāng děng fāng-jì zǔ-chéng, yòng yī fāng lái qū-chú fēng, hán, tán, shī yǐ-jí xiāo pǐ qù jì.

Qī-fāng shì fāng-jì zǔ-chéng de fǎ-zé zhī-yī. Chú-cǐ-yǐ-wài, hái-yǒu cóng zhì-liáo zuò-yòng lái fēn de. Rú zhāng jǐng-yuè céng bǎ fāng-jì fēn-wéi "bā-zhèn," jí bǔ-zhèn, hé-zhèn, gōng-zhèn, sàn-zhèn, hán-zhèn, rè-zhèn, gù-zhèn, yīn-zhèn. Bǔ-zhèn de fāng-jì shì yòng yú yuán-qì kuī-sǔn, tǐ-zhì xū-ruò de bìng-zhèng; hé-zhèn de fāng-jì shì yòng lái tiáo-he bìng-xié de piān-shèng; gōng-zhèn de fāng-jì shì yòng yú nèi-shí zhèng de; sàn-zhèn de fāng-jì shì yòng yú wài-gǎn zhèng de; hán-zhèn de fāng-jì shì yòng yú rè-zhèng de; rè-zhèn de fāng-jì shì yòng yú hán-zhèng de; gù-zhèn de fāng-jì shì yòng yú huá-xiè bù-jīn zhèng de; yīn-zhèn de fāng-jì dōu-shì yīn zhèng lì-fāng de.

Vocabulary 14.7

重复	chóng-fù	repeat; repetitive
五积散	wǔ-jī sǎn	powder for the five accumulations
桂枝汤	guì-zhī-tāng	decoction with guizhi
平胃散	píng-wèi-sǎn	powder calming down the stomach
二陈汤	èr-chén-tāng	decoction with two old (drugs)
痞	pǐ	block
除此以外	chú-cǐ-yǐ-wài	in addition
八阵	bā-zhèn	the eight strategic arrays
补阵	bǔ-zhèn	supplementing array
和阵	hé-zhèn	harmonizing array
攻阵	gōng-zhèn	attacking array
散阵	sàn-zhèn	dispersing array
寒阵	hán-zhèn	cooling array
热阵	rè-zhèn	heating array
固阵	gù-zhèn	consolidating array
因阵	yīn-zhèn	adapted array
亏损	kuī-sǔn	loss
偏胜	piān-shèng	unilateral dominance
内实	nèi-shí	internal repletion
滑泄	huá xiè	efflux diarrhea
立方	lì-fāng	set up a formula

Translation 14.7

7. The compound formula: "compound" is "complex" or "repetitive." Whenever an illness has comparatively many causes, or when the nature of an illness is comparatively complex, a compound formula must be employed for therapy. For example, the "powder for the five accumulations" is composed of the formulas "decoction with mahuang," "decoction with guizhi," "powder calming the stomach" and "decoction with

two old (drugs)." (These four formulas) are employed as one single formula to eliminate wind, cold, phlegm, and dampness, and also to dissolve blocks and to eliminate accumulations.

These seven formulas constitute one of the laws for the structuring of the prescriptions. In addition, there are (prescriptions) that are distinguished on the basis of their therapeutic functions. For example, Zhang Jingyue once differentiated the prescriptions as "eight strategic arrays," namely the array of supplementation, the array of harmonization, the array of attack, the array of supplementation, the array of harmonization, the array of attack, the array of dispersion, the array of cooling, the array of heating, the array of consolidation, and the array of adaptation. The prescriptions of the array of supplementation are used against pathoconditions of loss of original qi, of physical depletion, and weakness. The prescriptions of the array of harmonization are used to regulate a partial dominance of a pathogenic evil. The prescriptions of the array of attack are used against pathoconditions of internal repletion. The prescriptions of the array of dispersion are used against pathoconditions of exogenous affection. The prescriptions of the array of cooling are used against pathoconditions of heat. The prescriptions of the array of heating are used against pathoconditions of cold. The prescriptions of the array of consolidation are used against pathoconditions of efflux diarrhea that cannot be stopped. All the prescriptions of the array of adaptation are formulas set up adapted to the (respective) pathoconditions.

Text 14.8

中医的方剂，一般很难分类，原因是一个方剂往往包含多种效能，因而不能把它固定在一个门类内，即使几个方剂的治疗目的一致，但使用上又有很大出入。例如补养剂，不仅用于虚弱症，也能用于其他症候；而且补养一类的方剂也不是任何虚弱症都能适应的。此外，方剂中药物的加减，用量的多少，都能使其性质和作用改变。例如麻黄汤用麻黄，桂枝，杏仁，甘草组成，为发汗解表剂，倘把桂枝改为石膏，便为麻杏石甘汤，治肺热气喘，或把桂枝除去不用，便为三拗汤，治伤风感冒，鼻塞，咳嗽等症。

Transliteration 14.8

Zhōng-yī de fāng-jì, yī-bān hěn nán fēn-lèi, yuán-yīn shì yī ge fāng-jì wǎng-wǎng bāo-hán duō zhǒng xiào-néng, yīn-ér bù néng bǎ tā gù-dìng zài yī ge mén-lèi nèi, jí shǐ jǐ-ge fāng-jì de zhì-liáo mù-dì yī-zhì, dàn shǐ-yòng shàng yòu yǒu hěn dà chū-rù. Lì-rú bǔ-yǎng-jì, bù-jǐn yòng yú xū-ruò-zhèng, yě néng yòng yú qí-tā zhèng-hòu; ér-qiě bǔ-yǎng yī lèi de fāng-jì yě bù shì rèn-hé xū-ruò zhèng dōu néng shì-yìng de. Cǐ-wài, fāng-jì zhōng yào-wù de jiā-jiǎn, yòng liàng de duō-shǎo, dōu néng shǐ qí xìng-zhì hé zuò-yòng gǎi-biàn. Lì-rú má-huáng-tāng yòng má-huáng, guì-zhī, xìng-rén, gān-cǎo zǔ-chéng, wéi fā-hàn jiě-biǎo jì, tǎng bǎ guì-zhī gǎi-wéi shí-gāo, biàn wéi má-xìng-shí-gān-tāng, zhì fèi-rè qì-chuǎn, huò bǎ guì-zhī chú-qù-bù-yòng, biàn wéi sān-ǎo-tāng, zhì shāng-fēng gǎn-mào, bí-sè, ké-sòu děng zhèng.

Vocabulary 14.8

包含	bāo-hán	include
固定	gù-dìng	identify definitely
门类	mén-lèi	category
出入	chū-rù	difference
补养剂	bǔ-yǎng-jì	supplementing and nourishing prescription
适应	shì-yìng	be suited for
量	liàng	amount; dosage
甘草	gān-cǎo	(drug name) Glycyrrhiza uralensis Fisch.
倘 ... 便	tǎng ... biàn	if ..., then
改为	gǎi-wéi	replace by

石膏	shí-gāo	(drug name) gypsum
麻杏石甘汤	má-xìng-shí-gān-tāng	decoction with ma(huang), xing(ren), shi(gao) and gan(cao)
除去不用	chú-qù-bú-yòng	omit altogether
三拗汤	sān-ǎo-tāng	decoction with the three untreated (ingredients)

Translation 14.8

In general it is very difficult to categorize the prescriptions of Chinese medicine. The reason is that one single prescription often includes many types of usages. Hence it is impossible to identify them definitely as belonging to one single category. Even if the therapeutic objective of several prescriptions is identical, in their application there may be very significant differences nevertheless. For example, supplementing and nourishing prescriptions are used not only against pathoconditions of depletion and weakness, they may be used also against other pathoconditions. Also, prescriptions of the supplementing and nourishing type are not necessarily suited for (the treatment of) each and every pathocondition of depletion and weakness. Furthermore, when the drugs in a prescription are increased or decreased, and when the dosage applied is large or small, all this may change the nature and the function (of a prescription). For example, the "decoction with mahuang" is composed of mahuang, guizhi, xingren and gancao, and is a prescription to stimulate sweating and to open the outside (sections of the organism). When guizhi is replaced by shigao, (the "decoction with mahuang") becomes the "decoction with ma(huang), xing(ren), shi(gao) and gan(cao)," which cures lung heat and panting. Or, when guizhi is omitted altogether, (the "decoction with mahuang") becomes the "decoction with the three untreated (ingredients),"[1] which cures pathoconditions such as harm caused by wind, and common cold, congested nose, and cough.

Note

1 The name of this formula originates from the advice to decoct, in contrast to their usual processing, the three drugs used here as follows: mahuang with the knots of its stalks, xingren with the skin on the seed, and gancao in a raw or fresh state.

Text 15.1

方剂有多种剂型，各具不同的性质和不同的效用，常用的有丸，散，膏，丹，酒，汤等几类：

1. 丸剂：丸剂俗称丸药或药丸。将药物研成细粉后，加冷开水或蜜，或米糊，面糊等粘合物作成的圆形体。根据治疗上的要求，丸剂的大小和重量是不一致的，有小如芥子的，有大如弹丸的，也有如绿豆或梧桐子大的。大约大丸每粒重一钱，二钱或三钱；小丸每两二百至四百粒；细小丸每两六百至一千五百粒；极小丸每两五千至一万粒。丸药入胃，吸收较慢，多用于慢性疾病之须长期服食者。又病在下焦亦多用丸，取其吸收慢到达肠内才发生作用；也有急症，重症采用丸剂的，因可先期制成，取其便捷。

Transliteration 15.1

Fāng-jì yǒu duō zhǒng jì-xíng, gè jù bù-tóng de xìng-zhì hé bù-tóng de xiào-yòng, cháng-yòng de yǒu wán, sǎn, gāo, dān, jiǔ, tāng děng jǐ lèi:

1. Wán-jì: wán-jì sú-chēng wán-yào huò yào-wán. Jiāng yào-wù yán-chéng xì fěn hòu, jiā lěng kāi-shuǐ huò mì, huò mǐ-hú, miàn-hú děng nián-hé-wù zuò-chéng de yuán-xíng-tǐ. Gēn-jù zhì-liáo shàng-de yāo-qiú, wán-jì de dà-xiǎo hé zhòng-liàng shì bù yī-zhì de, yǒu xiǎo rú jiè-zǐ de, yǒu dà rú dàn-wán de, yě yǒu rú lǜ-dòu huò wú-tóng-zǐ dà de. Dà-yuē dà-wán měi lì zhòng yī qián, èr qián huò sān qián; xiǎo-wán měi liǎng èr-bǎi zhì sì-bǎi lì; xì-xiǎo-wán měi liǎng liù-bǎi zhì yī-qiān wǔ-bǎi lì; jí-xiǎo-wán měi liǎng wǔ-qiān zhì yī-wàn lì.

Wán-yào rù wèi, xī-shōu jiào màn, duō yòng yú màn-xìng jí-bìng zhī xū cháng-qī fú-shí zhě. Yòu bìng zài xià-jiāo yì duō yòng wán, qǔ-qí xī-shōu màn dào-dá cháng nèi cái fā-shēng zuò-yòng; yě yǒu jí-zhèng, zhòng-zhèng cǎi-yòng wán-jì de, yīn kě xiān-qī zhì-chéng, qǔ-qí biàn jié.

Vocabulary 15.1

剂型	jì-xíng	dosage form
具	jù	have
效用	xiào-yòng	effect
散	sǎn	powder
膏	gāo	paste
丹	dān	pellet; (a pellet-sized or powder preparation, sometimes produced by means of chemical processes)
酒	jiǔ	wine; liquor
丸剂	wán-jì	pill preparations
俗称	sú-chēng	be commonly called
丸药	wán-yào	pill drug
药丸	yào-wán	drug pill
研	yán	grind
研成	yán-chéng	grind into ...
粉	fěn	powder
开水	kāi-shuǐ	boiled water
蜜	mì	honey
米糊	mǐ-hú	rice paste
面糊	miàn-hú	flour paste
粘合物	nián-hé-wù	binder
作成	zuò-chéng	form to ...
圆形体	yuán-xíng-tǐ	round-shaped body
要求	yāo-qiú	requirement
重量	zhòng-liàng	weight
芥子	jiè-zǐ	mustard seed
弹丸	dàn-wán	bullet

绿豆	lǜ-dòu	green bean
梧桐子	wú-tóng-zǐ	wu tong seeds; seeds of Firmiana simplex (L.) W.F.Wight
大约	dà-yuē	in general
大丸	dà-wán	large pills
粒	lì	(measure word for pellets)
钱	qián	(weight; equal to 5 grams)
两	liǎng	(weight; equal to 50 grams)
小丸	xiǎo-wán	small pill
二百	èr-bǎi	two hundred
四百	sì-bǎi	four hundred
细小丸	xì-xiǎo-wán	very small pill
六百	liù-bǎi	six hundred
千	qiān	thousand
一千	yī-qiān	one thousand
五百	wǔ-bǎi	five hundred
极小丸	jí-xiǎo-wán	extremely small pill
五千	wǔ-qiān	five thousand
一万	yī-wàn	ten thousand
吸收	xī-shōu	absorb
服食	fú-shí	consume; take in (a medication)
取	qǔ	use
到达	dào-dá	reach
先期	xiān-qī	in advance
制成	zhì-chéng	prepare
捷	jié	quick

Translation 15.1

The prescriptions have many dosage forms, each of which possesses its individual character and its own effect. Commonly used types (of dosage forms) are pills, powders, pastes, pellets, wines, and decoctions.

1. Pill preparations: Pill preparations are commonly called "pill drugs" or "drug pills." After the drugs have been ground into a fine powder, (the pharmacist) adds binders such as cold boiled water, honey, rice paste or flour paste, and forms them to round-shaped bodies. In accordance with the requirements of the (respective) therapies, the size and the weight of the pills vary; some are small like mustard seeds, others are large like bullets. Still others have the size of green beans or wu tong seeds. In general, large pills have a weight of one, two, or three qian each; small pills amount from two hundred to four hundred per liang. Very small pills amount from six hundred to one thousand per liang, and extremely small pills amount from five thousand to ten thousand per liang.

Pill drugs enter the stomach, and their absorption is relatively slow. They are often used against chronic illnesses where they have to be consumed over an extended period of time. Also, when the illness is in the lower burner, pills are often used too, (an approach) taking advantage of (the phenomenon) that they develop their function only after they have been slowly absorbed into the intestines. Pill preparations are also used for violent pathoconditions, and against serious pathoconditions. Hence it is possible to prepare them in advance, and then take advantage of their convenient and quick (availability).

2.散剂：即粉剂，将药物研成细粉。有分研，合研，陆续配研等手续。一般多用合研，但带粘性的药物如乳香，没药，血竭，孩儿茶等，或挥发性强烈的药物如麝香，冰片，樟脑等；或较贵重的药物如犀角，羚羊角，珍珠，熊胆，蟾酥等，均用分研。陆续配研是因处方中含有少量贵重药或有其他必须分研的药物时用之，法将需要配研的药物分研后，置一种于乳钵内，然后加入等量的其它药粉，研匀以后，再加等量的其它药粉同研，陆续倍量，增加至全部混合均匀为止。

Transliteration 15.2

2. Sǎn-jì: jí fěn-jì, jiāng yào-wù yán-chéng xì fěn. Yǒu fēn-yán, hé-yán, lù-xù-pèi-yán děng shǒu-xù. Yī-bān duō yòng hé-yán, dàn dài-nián-xìng de yào-wù rú rǔ-xiāng, mò-yào, xuè-jié, hái-ér-chá děng, huò huī-fā-xìng qiáng-liè de yào-wù rú shè-xiāng, bīng-piàn, zhāng-nǎo děng; huò jiào guì-zhòng de yào-wù rú xī-jiǎo, líng-yáng-jiǎo, zhēn-zhū, xióng-dǎn, chán-sū děng, jūn yòng fēn-yán. Lù-xù-pèi-yán shì yīn chǔ-fāng zhōng hán-yǒu shǎo liàng guì-zhòng yào huò yǒu qí-tā bì-xū fēn-yán de yào-wù shí yòng zhī, fǎ jiāng xū-yào pèi-yán de yào-wù fēn-yán hòu, zhì yī zhǒng yú rǔ-bō nèi, rán-hòu jiā-rù děng-liàng de qí-tā yào-fěn, yán yún yǐ-hòu, zài jiā děng-liàng de qí-tā yào-fěn tóng yán, lù-xù bèi liàng, zēng-jiā zhì quán-bù hùn-hé jūn-yún wéi zhǐ.

Vocabulary 15.2

散剂	sǎn-jì	powder preparation
粉剂	fěn-jì	pulverized preparation
分研	fēn-yán	grind separately
合研	hé-yán	grind together
陆续	lù-xù	successive
陆续配研	lù-xù-pèi-yán	successively additive grinding
手续	shǒu-xù	procedure
带粘性	dài-nián-xìng	sticky
乳香	rǔ-xiāng	olibanum
没药	mò-yào	myrrha

血竭	xuè-jié	(drug name) Daemonorops draco Bl.; dragon's blood
孩儿茶	hái-ér-chá	catechu; (drug name) Acacia katechu (L.) Willd.
挥发性	huī-fā-xìng	volatile
强烈	qiáng-liè	strong
麝香	shè-xiāng	musk
冰片	bīng-piàn	borneol
樟脑	zhāng-nǎo	camphor
贵重	guì-zhòng	expensive
犀角	xī-jiǎo	rhinoceros horn
羚羊角	líng-yáng-jiǎo	antelope's horn
珍珠	zhēn-zhū	pearl
熊胆	xióng-dǎn	bear's gall
蟾酥	chán-sū	toad venom
配研	pèi-yán	grind while adding (individual substances)
置	zhì	bring; put
乳钵	rǔ-bō	mortar
等量	děng-liàng	equal amount
药粉	yào-fěn	drug powder
倍	bèi	double; multiply
混合	hùn-hé	mix
均匀	jūn-yún	evenly
至 ... 为止	zhì ... wéi zhǐ	until ...

Translation 15.2

2. Powder preparations: These are pulverized preparations; the drugs are ground into a fine powder. There are the different procedures of grinding (the drugs) separately, of grinding (the drugs) together, and of grinding while adding (the drugs) successively. In general, the grinding (of the drugs) together is used more often. However, sticky drugs such as olibanum, myrrh, dragon's blood, and catechu, or drugs with a strongly

developed volatile nature, such as musk, borneol, and camphor, or relatively expensive drugs such as rhinoceros horn, antelope's horn, pearls, bear's gall, and toad venom, are all ground separately. The grinding while adding (the drugs) successively is (carried out) because a prescription contains a small amount of precious drugs, or because there are other drugs that must be ground separately. The rule is (here) that once all the drugs that must be ground additively have been ground separately, one of them is brought into the mortar whereafter equal amounts of another drug powder are added. After these have been ground evenly, again an equal amount of another drug powder is added, whereafter (all powders in the mortar) are ground together. (This way) the amounts are multiplied successively, and the adding continues until the entire (prescription) has been mixed evenly.

3.膏剂：将药物用水煎汁，浓缩成稠厚半固体状，挑取适量，用开水冲服。一般制法，药物水浸一夜，煎两次至四次，取汁分次过滤，合并再熬，至不渗纸为度。另外有用植物油熬炼的，则为外贴用膏药。膏剂多为滋补类，用于慢性虚弱症，冬季服用的膏滋药亦属这一类。

4.丹剂：丹是用升华或熔合等方法制成的，主要为矿物类药物。也有用一般药物混合制成的。丹的剂型不一，有丸有散和锭剂等。用法与丸，散剂相同。

Transliteration 15.3

3. Gāo-jì: jiāng yào-wù yòng shuǐ jiān zhī, nóng-suō chéng chóu-hòu bàn-gù-tǐ zhuàng, tiāo-qǔ shí liàng, yòng kāi-shuǐ chòng-fú. Yī-bān zhì-fǎ, yào-wù shuǐ-jìn yī yè, jiān liǎng cì zhì sì cì, qǔ zhī fēn cì guò-lǜ, hé-bìng zài áo, zhì bù shèn zhǐ wéi dù. Lìng-wài yǒu yòng zhí-wù-yóu áo-liàn de, zé wéi wài tiē yòng gāo-yào.

Gāo-jì duō wéi zī-bǔ lèi, yòng yú màn-xìng xū-ruò zhèng, dōng-jì fú-yòng de gāo-zī-yào yì shǔ zhè yī lèi.

4. Dān-jì: dān shì yòng shēng-huá huò róng-hé děng fāng-fǎ zhì-chéng de, zhǔ-yào wéi kuàng-wù lèi yào-wù. Yě yǒu yòng yī-bān yào-wù hùn-hé zhì-chéng de. Dān de jì-xíng bù-yī, yǒu wán yǒu sǎn hé dìng-jì děng. Yòng-fǎ yǔ wán, sǎn-jì xiāng tóng.

Vocabulary 15.3

膏剂	gāo-jì	paste preparations
煎	jiān	boil (fast with strong heat)
汁	zhī	juice; extract
浓缩	nóng-suō	thicken by boiling; concentrate
稠厚	chóu-hòu	thick
半固体	bàn-gù-tǐ	semisolid
挑取	tiāo-qǔ	take
适	shì	suitable
冲服	chōng-fú	take in (with a liquid)

制法	zhì-fǎ	production method
水浸	shuǐ-jìn	soak in water
次	cì	-times
过滤	guò-lǜ	filtrate
合并	hé-bìng	combine
熬	áo	boil (slowly with gentle heat)
渗	shèn	seep
纸	zhǐ	paper
度	dù	degree
至 ... 为度	zhì ... wéi dù	until ...
另外	lìng-wài	in addition
植物油	zhí-wù-yóu	vegetable oil
熬炼	áo-liàn	boil
贴	tiē	paste
膏药	gāo-yào	paste drug
冬季	dōng-jì	winter
服用	fú-yòng	consume
膏滋药	gāo-zī-yào	pasty nutritious drug
丹剂	dān-jì	pellet preparation
升华	shēng-huá	sublimate
熔合	róng-hé	melt
矿物	kuàng-wù	mineral
锭剂	dìng-jì	ingot preparation

Translation 15.3

3. Paste preparations: the drugs are boiled with water (to generate an) extract. (This extract) is concentrated until it turns into a thick, semisolid consistency. Then a suitable amount (of this paste) is consumed together with boiled water. The common method to produce (such paste preparations) is to soak the drugs in water for one night, and then to boil this two to four times. Then the extract is filtrated several times (in separate portions. These portions are then) combined and boiled again until they (no longer) seep through paper. In addition, there are (paste

preparations) which are boiled with vegetable oil. They are applied externally as adhesive plasters.

Paste preparations are often nourishing (medications); they are employed against pathoconditions of chronic depletion and weakness. The pasty nutritious drugs consumed during winter belong to this category too.

4. Pellet preparations: Pellets are produced through procedures such as sublimation or melting; most important are mineral drugs. There are also (pellets) that are produced by combining common drugs. The dosage forms of pellets differ; they include pills, powders, and ingot preparations. The mode of application is identical with that of pills and powders.

Text 15.4

5. 酒剂：为药物用白酒作溶剂浸取所得的浸出液，故俗呼药酒。制法分冷浸和热浸两种，冷浸将药物泡在酒内，过一个时期即可服用；热浸是药物和酒密封坛内，隔水用文火缓缓加热，保持低温，经过三至七天，去火放冷。药酒多用于风湿痹痛，借酒的力量来帮助流通气血，加强舒筋活络的效能。

Transliteration 15.4

5. Jiǔ-jì: wéi yào-wù yòng bái-jiǔ zuò róng-jì jìn-qǔ suǒ dé de jìn-chū-yè, gù sú-hū yào-jiǔ. Zhì-fǎ fēn lěng-jìn hé rè-jìn liǎng zhǒng, lěng-jìn jiāng yào-wù pào zài jiǔ nèi, guò-yī-gè-shí-qī jí kě fú-yòng; rè-jìn shì yào-wù hé jiǔ mì-fēng tán nèi, gé shuǐ yòng wén-huǒ huǎn-huǎn jiā-rè, bǎo-chí dī wēn, jīng-guò sān zhì qī tiān, qù huǒ fàng lěng.

Yào-jiŭ duō yòng yú fēng-shī bì tòng, jiè jiŭ de lì-liàng lái bāng-zhù liú-tōng qì xuè, jiā-qiáng shū-jīn huó-luò de xiào-néng.

Vocabulary 15.4

酒剂	jiŭ-jì	alcoholic preparation
用 ... 作	yòng ... zuò ...	use .. for ...
白酒	bái-jiŭ	alcohol
溶剂	róng-jì	solvent
浸取	jìn-qŭ	soak and extract
浸出液	jìn-chū-yè	maceration liquid
俗呼	sú-hū	be commonly called
药酒	yào-jiŭ	medicinal wine
冷浸	lĕng-jìn	cold soaking
热浸	rè-jìn	hot soaking
泡	pào	steep
过一个时期	guò-yī-ge-shí-qī	after a (certain) time
密封	mì-fēng	thoroughly close
坛	tán	jar
文火	wén-huŏ	gentle fire
加热	jiā-rè	add heat; heat
去	qù	remove
放	fàng	let
痹	bì	stiffness
流	liú	flow
流通	liú-tōng	circulate; circulation
舒筋	shū-jīn	relax the sinews
活络	huó-luò	activate the network (vessels)

Translation 15.4

5. Alcoholic preparations: These are maceration liquids obtained by soaking and extracting drugs in alcohol as solvent. Hence they are commonly called "medicinal wines." The production methods are distinguished into the two types of cold soaking and hot soaking. Cold soaking is to steep the drugs in wine; after a (certain) time (the liquid) can be consumed. Hot soaking is to heat the drugs and the alcohol in a thoroughly closed jar over gentle fire, with (the jar) being separated by a water (bath from the source of the heat).[1] (The heat) is kept at a low temperature, and the fire is removed after three to seven days to let (the jar) cool down.

Medicinal wines are often employed against stiffness and pain in case of wind dampness. (Such therapies) make use here of the ability of alcohol to support the circulation of qi and blood, and to strengthen (drug) effects of sinew relaxation and network (vessel) activation.

Note

1 That is, the jar containing the drugs and the alcohol is not heated directly over the fire, but is placed into a large container that is filled with water and stands on the fire so that the heat reaches the jar only through the water. The jar must not touch the bottom in the water bath.

6. 汤剂：即水煎剂，用适当的水煎取药汁，倾出后加水再煎，第一次为头煎，第二次为二煎。一般每剂均煎两次，服法有头，二煎分开服的，也有将头，二煎药汁合并后，再分两次服的。临症上，汤剂应用最广，不仅吸取快，作用强，而且便于随症加减。丸，散，膏，丹和酒剂，多数属于成药，亦可视病症需要，处方配合。一部分丸散膏丹除单独使用外，也能放在汤剂内包煎，或用药汁冲服。

Transliteration 15.5

6. Tāng-jì: jí shuǐ jiān jì, yòng shì-dàng de shuǐ jiān qǔ yào-zhī, qīng-chū hòu jiā shuǐ zài jiān, dì-yī-cì wéi tóu-jiān, dì-èr-cì wéi èr-jiān. Yī-bān měi jì jūn jiān liǎng cì, fú-fǎ yǒu tóu, èr-jiān fēn-kāi fú de, yě yǒu jiāng tóu, èr-jiān yào-zhī hé-bìng hòu, zài fēn liǎng cì fú de.

Lín-zhèng shàng, tāng-jì yìng-yòng zuì guǎng, bù-jǐn xī-qǔ kuài, zuò-yòng qiáng, ér-qiě biàn yú suí zhèng jiā-jiǎn.

Wán, sǎn, gāo, dān hé jiǔ-jì, duō-shù shǔ-yú chéng-yào, yì kě shì bìng-zhèng xū-yào, chǔ-fāng pèi-hé. Yī bù-fèn wán sǎn gāo dān chú dān-dú shǐ-yòng wài, yě néng fàng zài tāng-jì nèi bāo jiān, huò yòng yào-zhī chōng-fú.

Vocabulary 15.5

汤剂	tāng-jì	decoction preparation
适当	shì-dàng	appropriate
药汁	yào-zhī	drug extract
倾出	qīng-chū	pour off
第一次	dì-yī-cì	the first time
头煎	tóu jiān	main boiling
第二次	dì-èr-cì	the second time
二煎	èr-jiān	the second boiling
服法	fú-fǎ	mode of intake
分开	fēn-kāi	separate; separately
服	fú	consume
吸取	xī-qǔ	absorb
多数	duō-shù	mostly
成药	chéng-yào	ready-made medication
视	shì	observe; behold
单独	dān-dú	individually
包	bāo	wrap

6. Decoction preparations: These are water-boiled decoctions. (The drugs) are boild with an appropriate (quantity of) water to obtain a drug extract. After pouring it off, water is added (again) and boiled a second time. The first time it is the main boiling; the second time it is the second boiling. In general, there are two boilings for each preparation. The modes of intake include consuming the main and the second boiling separately, but also mixing the drug extracts of the main and of the second boiling, and separating them again for consumption in two portions.

In clinical practice, decoction preparations are very widely applied. They are not only quickly absorbed, and their effects are strong, they are also easy to adapt to (individual) pathoconditions in that (their ingredients) are increased or decreased.

Pills, powders, pastes, pellets, and alcoholic preparations are mostly ready-made medications, but it is also possible to compose a prescription on the basis of the requirements of the pathoconditions of an illness. Some pills, powders, pastes, and pellets can be boiled, wrapped (in a clothbag), in decoctions, or may be taken combined with drug extracts, in addition to their independent application.

Text 15.6

中医的处方，实际上包括理，法，方，药一套知识在内，也就是理论和实践结合的具体表现。中医处方有一个特点，就是有案有方。案即脉案，处方时先将脉案写好，然后立方。脉案的内容包括症，因，脉，治四项，脉又包括四诊。一般先叙症状，次叙病因，次叙脉，舌，气色，最后指出治疗方针。当然，这也并不刻板，可以先叙症，脉，再叙因，治，或先把原因提出，再叙脉，症，只是大体上不越出这范围。

Transliteration 15.6

Zhōng-yī de chǔ-fāng, shí-jì-shàng bāo-kuò lǐ, fǎ, fāng, yào yī tào zhī-shí zài nèi, yě-jiù-shì lǐ-lùn hé shí-jiàn jié-hé de jù-tǐ biǎo-xiàn. Zhōng-yī chǔ-fāng yǒu yī ge tè-diǎn, jiù-shì yǒu àn yǒu fāng. Àn jí mài-àn, chǔ-fāng shí xiān jiāng mài-àn xiě hǎo, rán-hòu lì-fāng. Mài-àn de nèi-róng bāo-kuò zhèng, yīn, mài, zhì sì-xiàng, mài yòu bāo-kuò sì-zhěn. Yī-bān xiān xù zhèng-zhuàng, cì xù bìng-yīn, cì xù mài, shé, qì-sè, zuì-hòu zhǐ chū zhì-liáo fāng-zhēn. Dāng-rán, zhè yě bìng bù kè-bǎn, kě-yǐ xiān xù zhèng, mài, zài xù yīn, zhì, huò xiān bǎ yuán-yīn tí-chū, zài xù mài, zhèng, zhǐ shì dà-tǐ-shàng bù yuè-chū zhè fàn-wéi.

Vocabulary 15.6

包括 ... 在内	bāo-kuò ... zài nèi	include
理	lǐ	principle; theory
套	tào	(a totality of something that consists of individual parts)
知识	zhī-shí	knowledge
案	àn	case record
脉案	mài-àn	diagnostic record
写	xiě	write
好	hǎo	(particle indicating the conclusion of the activity or process signified by the immediately preceding verb)
叙	xù	assess
刻板	kè-bǎn	mechanical
只是	zhǐ-shì	it is just that
大体上	dà-tǐ-shàng	in general

Translation 15.6

In fact, the prescriptions of Chinese medicine include a whole (set of) knowledge (ranging from) theory and (therapy) patterns to prescriptions and drugs, and this is simply a manifestation of a combination of theory and practice. The prescriptions of Chinese medicine have a characteristic, that is, where there is a case record there is a prescription. By case record is meant the diagnostic record.[1] When (setting about the task of) making up a prescription, (a therapist) first completes writing down the diagnostic record, and then makes up the prescription. The contents of the diagnostic record include the four items pathoconditions, causes, pulse, and treatment; pulse includes (here) the four diagnostic (methods of looking, listening/smelling, asking, and feeling). In general, (a therapist) assesses the pathoconditions first, then he/she assesses the causes of the illness, then he/she assesses the (condition of the) pulse, the tongue, and the complexion, and at the very end he/she points out the principles of the treatment. That is, of course, not a mechanical (procedure); it may also be that the pathoconditions and the pulse are assessed first, and then the causes (of the illness), or that the causes are pointed out first, with pulse and pathoconditions being assessed later. It is just that on the whole (the procedure of making up prescriptions) does not leave this framework.

Note

1 The term *mai*, in general translatable as "vessel" or "pulse," is used here for diagnosis on the basis of signs which only the physician is trained to recognize and interpret.

对病症有了全面的认识之后，然后写方。写方时，哪些是主药，那些是协助的，胸中要有成竹。大概主药写在前，助药写在后，助药中又有主要和次要，同样依次书写，这就包含着君，臣，佐，使的意义在内。过去药方都直行写，习惯上分为三排，也有两排或四排的，视药味多少而定。先写第一排，再写第二，第三排。所以中药方应当一排一排看，如果一行一行看是分不出主次的。现在多数改用横写，比较以前更要清楚了。

Transliteration 15.7

Duì bìng-zhèng yǒu le quán-miàn de rèn-shi zhī hòu, rán-hòu xiě-fāng. Xiě-fāng shí, nà-xiē shì zhǔ-yào, nà-xiē shì xié-zhù de, xiōng-zhōng yào yǒu chéng-zhú. Dà-gài zhǔ-yào xiě zài qián, zhù-yào xiě zài hòu, zhù-yào zhōng yòu yǒu zhǔ-yào hé cì-yào, tóng-yàng yī-cì shū-xiě, zhè jiù bāo-hán zhe jūn, chén, zuǒ, shǐ de yì-yì zài nèi. Guò-qù yào-fāng dōu zhí háng xiě, xí-guàn-shang fēn-wéi sān pái, yě yǒu liǎng pái huò sì pái de, shì yào-wèi duō-shǎo ér dìng. Xiān xiě dì yī pái, zài xiě dì èr, dì sān pái. Suǒ-yǐ zhōng-yào-fāng yīng-dāng yī-pái-yī-pái kàn, rú-guǒ yī-háng-yī-háng kàn shì fēn-bù-chū zhǔ cì de. Xiàn-zài duō-shù gǎi yòng héng xiě, bǐ-jiào yǐ-qián gèng yào qīng-chu le.

Vocabulary 15.7

写方	xiě-fāng	write out a prescription
哪些	nǎ-xiē	which
胸中有	xiōng-zhōng yǒu	have in mind
成竹	chéng-zhú	the complete bamboo (a metaphor taken from painting, indicating a well-thought-out plan)
大概	dà-gài	as a rule; most likely
助药	zhù-yào	supporting drug
依次	yī-cì	in succession; in proper order; one after another
书写	shū-xiě	write down
过去	guò-qù	earlier; formerly
行	háng	column
习惯上	xí-guàn-shàng	traditionally; usually
排	pái	line
视 ... 而定	shì ... ér dìng	determine on the basis of ...
药味	yào-wèi	medicinal drug

中药方	zhōng-yào-fāng	prescription of Chinese drugs; Chinese pharmaceutical prescriptions
一排一排	yī-pái-yī-pái	line after line
一行一行	yī-háng-yī-háng	column after column
分不出	fēn-bù-chū	impossible to distinguish
现在	xiàn-zài	now
改	gǎi	change
用	yòng	with ... (+ verb)
比较	bǐ-jiào	compare with
要	yào	certainly; definitely

Translation 15.7

Once a complete understanding of an illness and (its) pathoconditions has been obtained, a prescription is written out. When writing out a prescription, it is necessary to have a well-thought-out plan of which (drugs) will be the main drugs, and which will be the supporters. Most likely the main drugs will be written at the beginning (of the prescription), and the supporting drugs at the end. Among the supporting drugs are, once again, those of primary importance, and others of secondary importance. They are written down in proper order in the same manner. This then includes the meaning of ruler, minister, assistant, and messenger. Formerly, drug prescriptions were always written in vertical columns, and they were customarily divided into three lines. There were also two line or four line (prescriptions, the number of lines) being determined in accordance with the number of drugs (prescribed). The first line was written first, then the second and the third lines. Hence the prescriptions of Chinese pharmaceutics had to be read line after line; if read column after column it was impossible to distinguish between main (drugs) and secondary (drugs). Unlike (before), nowadays (therapists) mostly write in horizontal (lines). In comparison with the past, this is certainly clearer.

Text 15.8

研究处方，必须多看医案，医案是中医的临症记录，如"临症指南"就是叶天士的医案，也就是他平日治病的方案。由于中医处方不只记录用药，更全面地记录下有关病人的得病原因，症状，四诊，治法，处方，和详细的分析，论断。是理论与实践相结合的产物，对学习具有很大的帮助和启发作用。同时一个人的见解和经验毕竟有限，还必须广泛地多看各家医案，虽然不一定都有好处，但必然有其特长的地方，我们认为只有象蜜蜂酿蜜般的吸取百花精华，才能更丰富自己的知识和经验。因此，也能说各家医案是医生终身的良师。

Transliteration 15.8

Yán-jiū chǔ-fāng, bì-xū duō kàn yī-àn, yī-àn shì zhōng-yī de lín-zhèng jì-lù, rú "lín-zhèng-zhǐ-nán" jiù-shì yè tiān-shì de yī-àn, yě-jiù-shì tā píng-rì zhì-bìng de fāng-àn. Yóu-yú zhōng-yī chǔ-fāng bù zhǐ jì-lù yòng yào, gèng quán-miàn de jì-lù-xià yǒu-guān bìng-rén de dé bìng yuán-yīn, zhèng-zhuàng, sì-zhěn, zhì-fǎ, chǔ-fāng, hé xiáng-xì de fēn-xī, lùn-duàn. Shì lǐ-lùn yǔ shí-jiàn xiāng jié-hé de chǎn-wù, duì xué-xí jù-yǒu hěn dà de bāng-zhù hé qǐ-fā zuò-yòng. Tóng-shí yī ge rén de jiàn-jiě hé jīng-yàn bì-jìng yǒu-xiàn, hái bì-xū guǎng-fàn de duō kàn gè jiā yī-àn, suī-rán bù-yī-dìng dōu yǒu hǎo-chù, dàn bì-rán yǒu qí tè-cháng de dì-fāng, wǒ-men rèn-wéi zhǐ yǒu xiàng mì-fēng niàng mì bān de xī-qǔ bǎi huā jīng-huá, cái néng gèng fēng-fù zì-jǐ de zhī-shí hé jīng-yàn. Yīn-cǐ, yě néng shuō gè jiā yī-àn shì yī-shēng zhōng-shēn de liáng shī.

Vocabulary 15.8

医案	yī-àn	medical case histories
记录	jì-lù	record
临症指南	lín-zhèng-zhǐ-nán	(book title) "Clinical Guideline"
叶天士	yè tiān-shì	(author's name) Ye Tianshi
他	tā	he/she; his/her
平日	píng-rì	daily

方案	fāng-àn	program
记录下	jì-lù-xià	record; write down
论断	lùn-duàn	evaluation
产物	chǎn-wù	product
启发	qǐ-fā	enlighten
见解	jiàn-jiě	perspective
经验	jīng-yàn	experience
有限	yǒu-xiàn	limited
家	jiā	expert; author
好处	hǎo-chù	benefit; advantage
必然	bì-rán	definitely
蜜蜂	mì-fēng	bee
酿	niàng	produce
般	bān	kind; type
花	huā	flower
丰富	fēng-fù	rich
自己	zì-jǐ	self; own
终身	zhōng-shēn	the entire life
师	shī	teacher

Translation 15.8

(Those who) study how to write out prescriptions, should frequently read medical case histories. Medical case histories are the clinical records of Chinese medicine. For example, the *Lin zheng zhi nan* consists of the case histories (documented) by Ye Tianshi,[1] and at the same time it contains the program of his daily therapies. Because the prescriptions of Chinese medicine do not only record the use of drugs, they are even more complete in that they record with respect to the patient the reasons why he/she got the illness, the pathoconditions, the (results of the) four examinations, the therapeutic pattern, and the prescription, as well as a detailed analysis and evaluation (of the case at hand). (Such medical case histories) are a product of a combination of theory and practice; they are very helpful and have an enlightening function for (practical) studies. At the same time (it should be pointed out that) a single person's perspective and experience are limited; in addition (to the clinical records of Ye Tianshi students) should widely read many authors' case histories. Even though they are not necessarily all of use, they nevertheless all have their respective strong points. We believe that only if (therapists) draw the essence of a hundred flowers like the bees do when they make honey, (they) will be able to further enrich (their) knowledge and experience. Hence (we) may also say that any author's case histories are good teachers for a physician's entire life.

Note

1 Ye Gui 叶桂 (Tianshi) (1667-1746) was a famous physician and author.

LESSON 16: THE PREPARATION OF DRUGS

Text 16.1

药物的产地和采集时期，对于疗效有着密切关系。举例来说，如贝母产于四川的和浙江的效用不同。因而，中药有很多名字是根据产地而起的，如党参因产上党得名，川芎因产四川得名。在一般处方上还特地写明产地如川贝母，浙贝母，以及川桂枝，川黄柏，广木香，云茯苓，建泽泻等，目前有些已不需要，有些还是应当写明。由于植物的生长成熟各有一定时期，所以药物气味的保全和消失，全靠采集季节的是否适当，及时采集不仅提高功效，还能保证丰收。

Transliteration 16.1

Yào-wù de chǎn-dì hé cǎi-jí-shí-qī, duì-yú liáo-xiào yǒu zhe mì-qiè guān-xi. Jǔ-lì-lái shuō, rú bèi-mǔ chǎn yú sì-chuān de hé zhè-jiāng de xiào-yòng bù-tóng. Yīn-ér, zhōng-yào yǒu hěn duō míng-zì shì gēn-jù chǎn-dì ér qǐ de, rú dǎng-shēn yīn chǎn shàng-dǎng dé míng, chuān-xiōng yīn chǎn sì-chuān dé míng. Zài yī-bān chǔ-fāng shàng hái tè de xiě-míng chǎn-dì rú chuān-bèi-mǔ, zhè-bèi-mǔ, yǐ-jí chuān-guì-zhī, chuān-huáng-bò, guǎng-mù-xiāng, yún-fú-líng, jiàn-zé-xiè děng, mù-qián yǒu xiē yǐ bù xū-yào, yǒu xiē hái-shì yīng-dāng xiě-míng.

Yóu-yú zhí-wù de shēng-zhǎng chéng-shú gè yǒu yī-dìng shí-qī, suǒ-yǐ yào-wù qì-wèi de bǎo-quán hé xiāo-shī, quán kào cǎi-jí jì-jié de shì-fǒu shì-dāng, jí-shí cǎi-jí bù-jǐn tí-gāo gōng-xiào, hái néng bǎo-zhèng fēng shōu.

Vocabulary 16.1

产地	chǎn-dì	place of production; place of origin
采集时期	cǎi-jí-shí-qī	time of collection
贝母	bèi-mǔ	(drug name) Fritillaria cirrhosa D. Don.
四川	sì-chuān	(name of province) Sichuan
浙江	zhè-jiāng	(name of province) Zhejiang
名字	míng-zì	name; designation
党参	dǎng-shēn	(drug name) Codonopsis pilosula (Franch.) Nannf.

上党	shàng-dǎng	(place name) Shangdang
川芎	chuān-xiōng	(drug name) Ligusticum wallichii Franch.
特	tè	special
写明	xiě-míng	write out; adduce
川贝母	chuān-bèi-mǔ	(the drug) beimu from (the province of Si)chuan
浙贝母	zhè-bèi-mǔ	(the drug) beimu from (the province of Zhe)jiang
川桂枝	chuān-guì-zhī	(the drug) guizhi from (the province of Si)chuan
川黄柏	chuān-huáng-bò	(the drug) huangbo from (the province of Si)chuan
广木香	guǎng-mù-xiāng	(the drug) muxiang from (the province of) Guang(dong)
云茯苓	yún-fú-líng	(the drug) fuling from (the province of) Yun(nan)
建泽泻	jiàn-zé-xiè	(the drug) zexie from (the province of Fu)jian
目前	mù-qián	today; at present
还是	hái-shì	still
植物	zhí-wù	plant
成熟	chéng-shú	maturing
保全	bǎo-quán	preserve
全	quán	total
采集	cǎi-jí	collect; harvest; gather
提高	tí-gāo	increase
功效	gōng-xiào	efficacy
保证	bǎo-zhèng	guarantee
丰	fēng	rich

Translation 16.1

The places of origin and the times of collection of drugs are closely related to their therapeutic efficacy. For example, the effects of beimu grown in Sichuan and (of beimu grown) in Zhejiang are different. Hence in Chinese pharmaceutics there are very many names (of drugs) that have their origin in the places of growth (of the respective substances). Examples are dangshen which has its name because it is a product of Shangdang, or chuanxiong which has its name because it is a product of Sichuan. Even in a common prescription the names of the place of origin are specified, such as (Si)chuan beimu, and (Zhe)jiang beimu, as well as (Si)chuan guizhi, (Si)chuan huangbo, (Guang)dong muxiang, (Yun)nan fuling, and (Fu)jian zexie. Today some such (designations) are no longer necessary, while there are others that should still be specified.

Because the growth and the maturing of plants is tied to fixed time periods, preservation and loss of the qi and of the flavor of the drugs depend entirely on whether the season during which they were gathered was appropriate or not. To gather (drugs) in time not only increases their efficacy, it also guarantees a good harvest.

生药中有些具有毒性，或性质猛烈，不能直接服用；有些气味恶劣，不利于服用；有些必须除去不适用部分；也有些生和熟的作用有差别。因此，中药里有很多是经过加工的。对药物加工的意义，不外消除或减低药物的毒性，以及适当地改善药物性能。前者如半夏，用生的，会刺激咽喉，使人音哑或中毒，须用姜汁制过；后者如地黄，用生的，性寒，能凉血，蒸制成为熟地，其性就变为温而补血；或将生地炒炭则止血，熟地炒松则可减少粘腻的流弊。中药加工，称做炮制，也叫修治。

Transliteration 16.2

Shēng-yào zhōng yǒu xiē jù-yǒu dú-xìng, huò xìng-zhì měng-liè, bù néng zhí-jiē fú-yòng; yǒu xiē qì-wèi è-liè, bù lì yú fú-yòng; yǒu xiē bì-xū chú-qù bù shì-yòng bù-fèn; yě yǒu xiē shēng hé shú de zuò-yòng yǒu chā-bié. Yīn-cǐ, zhōng-yào lǐ yǒu hěn duō shì jīng-guò jiā-gōng de. Duì yào-wù jiā-gōng de yì-yì, bù wài xiāo-chú huò jiǎn-dī yào-wù de dú-xìng, yǐ-jí shì-dàng de gǎi-shàn yào-wù-xìng-néng. Qián zhě rú bàn-xià, yòng shēng de, huì cì-jī yān-hóu, shǐ rén yīn-yǎ huò zhòng-dú, xū yòng jiāng-zhī zhì-guò; hòu zhě rú dì-huáng, yòng shēng de, xìng hán, néng liáng xuè, zhēng-zhì chéng-wéi shú-dì, qí xìng jiù biàn-wéi wēn ér bǔ-xuè; huò jiāng shēng-dì chǎo-tàn zé zhǐ-xuè, shú-dì chǎo sōng zé kě jiǎn-shǎo nián-nì de liú-bì. Zhōng-yào jiā-gōng, chēng-zuò páo-zhì, yě jiào xiū-zhì.

Vocabulary 16.2

生	shēng	raw
生药	shēng-yào	raw drug
恶劣	è-liè	vile; foul
不利于	bù-lì-yú	not conducive to
除去	chú-qù	discard
适用	shì-yòng	suitable
熟	shú	processed
加工	jiā-gōng	process
消除	xiāo-chú	eliminate
减低	jiǎn-dī	reduce
药物性能	yào-wù-xìng-néng	drug ability

半夏	bàn-xià	(drug name) Pinellia ternata (Thub.) Breit.
音哑	yīn-yǎ	loss of voice
姜汁	jiāng-zhī	ginger extract
制	zhì	control; check; process
制过	zhì-guò	control drawbacks
蒸	zhēng	steam
蒸制	zhēng-zhì	process by steaming
熟地	shú-dì	(drug name) Rehmannia glutinosa (Gaertn.) Libosch.
变为	biàn-wéi	change to
炒	chǎo	fry
炭	tàn	coal
炮制	páo-zhì	process by roasting (general designation of the pharmaceutical processing of Chinese drugs)
修治	xiū-zhì	trim and manage (general designation of the pharmaceutical processing of Chinese drugs)

Translation 16.2

Among the raw drugs are some that have a toxic nature, and others whose character is violent; they cannot be taken right away. There are some whose qi and flavor are foul; they are not conducive to intake. There are some where unsuitable parts must be discarded; and there are some where the effects of a raw state and of a processed state are different. Hence in Chinese pharmaceutics there are very many (drugs) that have been subjected to processing. The significance of drug processing lies in an elimination or reduction of a toxic character of a drug, and in an appropriate improvement of a drugs's abilities. An example of the former is banxia. If used raw, it may irritate the throat, and cause loss of voice or poisoning. It is necessary to use ginger juice to control these drawbacks. An example of the latter is dihuang. If used in a raw state, its nature is cold, and it may cool the blood. Through steam processing it is transformed into shudi(huang, a drug) whose nature has changed to warm, and which may supplement the blood. Or, if raw di(huang) is fried to charcoal, then it stops bleeding. If shudi(huang) is fried until it is crisp, then this decreases its disadvantage of being a sticky (substance). Processing in Chinese pharmaceutics is called paozhi, and it is also called xiuzhi.

Text 16.3

炮制时有用酒，醋，盐水等配合者，这是根据治疗的需要。如酒制取其升提，姜汁制取其发散，盐水制取其入肾而软坚，醋制取其走肝而收敛，童便制取其清火下降，米泔制取其润燥和中，乳汁制取其润枯生血，蜂蜜制取其甘缓补脾。还有用土炒取其走中焦，用黑豆，甘草汤浸泡取其解毒。这些都是前人的经验，现在仍旧沿用。

Transliteration 16.3

Páo-zhì shí yǒu yòng jiǔ, cù, yán-shuǐ děng pèi-hé zhě, zhè shì gēn-jù zhì-liáo de xū-yào. Rú jiǔ-zhì qǔ qí shēng-tí, jiāng-zhī-zhì qǔ qí fā-sàn, yán-shuǐ-zhì qǔ qí rù shèn ér ruǎn jiān, cù-zhì qǔ qí zǒu gān ér shōu-liǎn, tóng-biàn-zhì qǔ qí qīng huǒ xià-jiàng, mǐ-gān-zhì qǔ qí rùn zào hé zhōng, rǔ-zhī-zhì qǔ qí rùn kū shēng xuè, fēng-mì-zhì qǔ qí gān huǎn bǔ pí. Hái-yǒu yòng tǔ chǎo qǔ qí zǒu zhōng-jiāo, yòng hēi-dòu, gān-cǎo tāng jìn-pào qǔ qí jiě-dú. Zhè-xiē dōu shì qián-rén de jīng-yàn, xiàn-zài réng-jiù yán-yòng.

Vocabulary 16.3

醋	cù	vinegar
盐水	yán-shuǐ	brine
酒制	jiǔ-zhì	processing with alcohol
升提	shēng-tí	rise
姜汁制	jiāng-zhī-zhì	processing with ginger extract
发散	fā-sàn	disperse
盐水制	yán-shuǐ-zhì	processing with brine
醋制	cù-zhì	processing with vinegar
收敛	shōu-liǎn	draw together; contract
童便制	tóng-biàn-zhì	processing with boys' urine
下降	xià-jiàng	descend
米泔制	mǐ-gān-zhì	processing with water used for washing rice
乳汁制	rǔ-zhī-zhì	processing with milk
蜂蜜制	fēng-mì-zhì	processing with honey
黑豆	hēi-dòu	black soybean
浸泡	jìn-pào	soak
仍旧	réng-jiù	as before; unchanged
沿用	yán-yòng	remain in use

Translation 16.3

Whether wine, vinegar, or brine is used in processing depends on the requirements of the therapy. For example, in processing (a drug) with wine advantage is taken of (the alcohol's) rising (nature). If (a drug) is treated with ginger extract, advantage is taken of its dispersing (nature).

If (a drug) is treated with brine, use is made of its (ability to) enter the kidneys and to soften what is hard. If (a drug) is treated with vinegar, advantage is taken of its (ability to) enter the liver and to draw together what has gone asunder. If (a drug) is treated with boys' urine, advantage is taken of its (ability to) cool the fire and to descend. If (a drug) is treated with water in which rice has been washed, advantage is taken of its (ability to) moisten what is dry, and to harmonize the (body's) center. If (a drug) is treated with (women's) milk, advantage is taken of its (ability to) moisten what is whithered, and to generate blood. And if (a drug) is treated with honey, advantage is taken of its sweet and relaxing (nature, and of its ability to) supplement the spleen. Also, (drugs) may be fried in soil, which is to take advantage of the latter's (ability to) enter the central burner. (Furthermore, drugs) may be soaked in decoctions of black soybeans or gancao, which is to take advantage of their (ability to) dissolve poison. All these are experiences of people of former times that have remained in use until today.

Text 16.4

研究药物当以功效为主，然而，更重要的一面，是必须研究其药理作用。中医对于药理的研究，采用阴阳，五行学说来区别药物的性能，分为气和味两大类。疾病的产生，不论外因或内因引起，均使体内脏气偏盛偏衰，因药物的气味也各有偏胜，故可借药物的偏胜之气来纠正病体的偏盛偏衰。比如热病用寒性药来治，寒病用热性药来治，体虚用补药，病实用泻药，都是利用药物的偏胜来调整病体的偏盛偏衰，也就是以偏救偏。

Transliteration 16.4

Yán-jiū yào-wù dāng yǐ gōng-xiào wéi zhǔ, rán-ér, gèng zhòng-yào de yī miàn, shì bì-xū yán-jiū qí yào-lǐ-zuò-yòng. Zhōng-yī duì-yú yào-lǐ de yán-jiū, cǎi-yòng yīn yáng, wǔ-xíng xué-shuō lái qū-bié yào-wù de xìng-néng, fēn-wéi qì hé wèi liǎng dà lèi. Jí-bìng de chǎn-shēng, bù-lùn wài-yīn huò nèi-yīn yǐn-qǐ, jūn shì tǐ-nèi zàng-qì piān-shèng piān-shuāi, yīn yào-wù de qì-wèi yě gè yǒu piān-shèng, gù kě jiè yào-wù de piān-shèng zhī qì lái jiū-zhèng bìng-tǐ de piān-shèng piān-shuāi. Bǐ-rú rè-bìng yòng hán-xìng-yào lái zhì, hán-bìng yòng rè-xìng-yào lái zhì, tǐ xū yòng bǔ-yào, bìng shí yòng xiè-yào, dōu shì lì-yòng yào-wù de piān-shèng lái tiáo-zhěng bìng-tǐ de piān-shèng piān-shuāi, yě-jiù-shì yǐ-piān-jiù-piān.

Vocabulary 16.4

然而	rán-ér	still; however
药理作用	yào-lǐ-zuò-yòng	pharmacological effect
药理	yào-lǐ	principles of drug (effects)
性能	xìng-néng	ability; effect
偏盛	piān-shèng	unilateral flourishing
偏衰	piān-shuāi	unilaterial weakness
纠正	jiū-zhèng	correct
寒性药	hán-xìng-yào	drug of cold nature
寒病	hán-bìng	cold illness
热性药	rè-xìng-yào	drug of hot nature
补药	bǔ-yào	supplementing drug
调整	tiáo-zhěng	regulate
以偏救偏	yǐ-piān-jiù-piān	save the unilateral with the unilateral

Translation 16.4

The study of drugs should emphasize their effects. Still, an even more important aspect lies in the necessity to study their pharmacological functions. In its study of the principles of drug (effects), Chinese medicine uses the theories of yinyang and of the five phases to distinguish the effects of the drugs, and to classify them according to the two major categories of qi and flavor. Whenever an illness emerges, no matter whether it was stimulated through an exogenous cause or through an internal cause, in all cases this leads to a unilateral flourishing or weakness of visceral qi inside the body. Because the qi and the flavors of drugs are similarly unilaterally dominant, it is possible to take advantage of this unilaterally dominating qi of drugs to correct the unilateral flourishing or unilateral weakness of the sick body. For example, in case of a heat illness drugs of a cold nature are used for treatment, and in case of a cold illness drugs of a hot nature are used for treatment. If the body is depleted, supplementing drugs are used; if (a person) suffers from repletion, draining drugs are used. In all cases the unilateral dominance (of a nature) in a drug is used to regulate the unilateral flourishing or unilateral weakness of the sick body. That is, the unilaterial is saved with the unilateral.

1. 气：药性的气分为四种，即寒，热，温，凉。四种之外，还有平气。所谓平气，实际上仍然偏温或偏凉，不过性质比较和平不太显著而已，故一般称为四气。寒，热，温，凉四种不同的药性，可以分作两面来看，热性和寒性是两个极端，温次于热，凉次于寒，故细致地说，有寒性药，凉性药和热性药，温性药，也可简单地说成寒凉药和温热药。把药物分为四气，是就药物作用于人体所引起的各种反应中归纳出来的，也是药物性能的概括。例如石膏，知母等能治疗热病，便知其有寒凉性质；附子，肉桂等能治疗寒病，便知其有温热性质。也就是寒性和凉性药，具有清热，泻火作用；热性药和温性药具有祛寒，回阳作用。

Transliteration 16.5

1. Qì: yào-xìng de qì fēn-wéi sì zhǒng, jí hán, rè, wēn, liáng. Sì zhǒng zhī wài, hái-yǒu píng-qì. Suǒ-wèi píng-qì, shí-jì-shàng réng-rán piān-wēn huò piān-liáng, bù-guò xìng-zhì bǐ-jiào hé-píng bù tài xiǎn-zhù ér-yǐ, gù yī-bān chēng-wéi sì-qì.

Hán, rè, wēn, liáng sì zhǒng bù-tóng de yào-xìng, kě-yǐ fēn-zuò liǎng miàn lái kàn, rè-xìng hé hán-xìng shì liǎng ge jí-duān, wēn cì yú rè, liáng cì yú hán, gù xì-zhì-de-shuō, yǒu hán-xìng-yào, liáng-xìng-yào hé rè-xìng-yào, wēn-xìng-yào, yě kě jiǎn-dān de shuō-chéng hán-liáng-yào hé wēn-rè-yào. Bǎ yào-wù fēn-wéi sì-qì, shì jiù yào-wù zuò-yòng yú rén-tǐ suǒ yǐn-qǐ de gè zhǒng fǎn-yìng zhōng guī-nà chū-lái de, yě shì yào-wù xìng-néng de gài-kuò. Lì-rú shí-gāo, zhī-mǔ děng néng zhì-liáo rè-bìng, biàn zhī qí yǒu hán-liáng xìng-zhì; fù-zǐ, ròu-guì děng néng zhì-liáo hán-bìng, biàn zhī qí yǒu wēn-rè xìng-zhì. Yě-jiù-shì hán-xìng hé liáng-xìng-yào, jù-yǒu qīng rè, xiè huǒ zuò-yòng; rè-xìng-yào hé wēn-xìng-yào jù-yǒu qū hán, huí-yáng zuò-yòng.

Vocabulary 16.5

平气	píng-qì	balanced qi
偏温	piān-wēn	unilaterally warm (qi)
偏凉	piān-liáng	unilaterally cool (qi)
四气	sì-qì	the four qi
极端	jí-duān	extreme
次于	cì yú	be secondary to
细致地说	xì-zhì-de-shuō	strictly speaking; looked at in detail
凉性药	liáng-xìng-yào	drug of cool nature
温性药	wēn-xìng-yào	drug of warm nature
说成	shuō-chéng	designate as; speak of
寒凉药	hán-liáng-yào	cold-cool drug
温热药	wēn-rè-yào	warm-hot drug
概括	gài-kuò	outline
知母	zhī-mǔ	(drug name) Anemarrhena asphodeloides Bge.
凉性	liáng-xìng	cool nature

Translation 16.5

1. Qi: In the nature of the drugs (Chinese medicine) distinguishes among four types of qi, namely cold, hot, warm, and cool (qi). In addition to these four types there is the balanced qi. In reality, this so-called balanced qi is nevertheless a unilaterally warm or unilaterally cool (qi); however, its character is relatively harmonious and not overly notable. Hence in general (Chinese medicine) speaks of the four qi.

Cold, hot, warm, and cool, the four types of different drug natures, may be seen in two perspectives. Hot nature and cold nature are two extremes. Warmth is secondary to heat; coolness is secondary to cold. Hence, looked at in detail, there are drugs of cold nature, and there are drugs of cool nature, there are drugs of hot nature, and there are drugs of warm nature. But it is also possible to simply speak of cold-cool drugs and of warm-hot drugs. The differentiation of drugs according to the four qi has been concluded inductively from the various reactions called forth in the human body by the effects of drugs; it is also an outline of the abilities of the drugs. For example, shigao and zhimu can cure heat illnesses; hence (we) know of their cold-cool nature. Fuzi and rougui can cure cold illnesses; hence (we) know of their warm-hot nature. That is to say, drugs of cold nature and of a cool nature possess the effects of cooling heat and of draining fire. Drugs of a hot nature and drugs of a warm nature possess the effects of eliminating cold and make the yang return.

2. 味：味分五味；就是酸，苦，甘，辛，咸。前人通过亲自尝试的办法辨认药味，在长期实践中逐渐认识到药物具有各种味道，因而具有各种不同的性能，内经所说的辛散，酸收，甘缓，苦坚，咸软，便是把五味的作用进行了归纳。在这基础上，前人又补充为：辛味能散能行，酸味能收能涩，甘味能补能和，苦味能燥能泻，咸味能软能下。五味与五行的配合是：酸属木，苦属火，甘属土，辛属金，咸属水。因而五味与五脏的关系是：酸入肝，苦入心，甘入脾，辛入肺，咸入肾。然而，五味和上面所说的四气一样，其性皆偏，它能调整脏气的不平，也能伤害脏气而造成疾病。

Transliteration 16.6

2. Wèi: wèi fēn wǔ-wèi; jiù-shì suān, kǔ, gān, xīn, xián. Qián-rén tōng-guò qīn-zì cháng-shì de bàn-fǎ biàn-rèn yào-wèi, zài cháng-qī shí-jiàn zhōng zhú-jiàn rèn-shi-dào yào-wù jù-yǒu gè zhǒng wèi-dào, yīn-ér jù-yǒu gè zhǒng bù-tóng de xìng-néng, nèi-jīng suǒ-shuō-de xīn sàn, suān shōu, gān huǎn, kǔ jiān, xián ruǎn, biàn shì bǎ wǔ-wèi de zuò-yòng jìn-xíng le guī-nà. Zài zhè jī-chǔ shàng, qián-rén yòu bǔ-chōng wéi: xīn-wèi néng sàn néng xíng, suān-wèi néng shōu néng sè, gān-wèi néng bǔ néng hé, kǔ-wèi néng zào néng xiè, xián-wèi néng ruǎn néng xià.

Wǔ-wèi yǔ wǔ-xíng de pèi-hé shì: suān shǔ mù, kǔ shǔ huǒ, gān shǔ tǔ, xīn shǔ jīn, xián shǔ shuǐ. Yīn-ér wǔ-wèi yǔ wǔ-zàng de guān-xi shì: suān rù gān, kǔ rù xīn, gān rù pí, xīn rù fèi, xián rù shèn. Rán-ér, wǔ-wèi hé shàng-miàn suǒ-shuō-de sì-qì yī-yàng, qí xìng jiē piān, tā néng tiáo-zhěng zàng-qì de bù-píng, yě néng shāng-hài zàng-qì ér zào-chéng jí-bìng.

Vocabulary 16.6

五味	wǔ-wèi	the five flavors
通过	tōng-guò	by way of
亲自	qīn-zì	personal
尝试	cháng-shì	test; taste
辨认	biàn-rèn	distinguish
认识到	rèn-shi-dào	realize; recognize
味道	wèi-dào	flavor
辛味	xīn-wèi	acrid flavor
酸味	suān-wèi	sour flavor
甘味	gān-wèi	sweet flavor
苦味	kǔ-wèi	bitter flavor
咸味	xián-wèi	salty flavor
不平	bù-píng	imbalance

Translation 16.6

2. Flavor: The flavors are distinguished into the five flavors; these are sour, bitter, sweet, acrid, and salty. By way of personally tasting (the drugs), the people of former times have distinguished the drug flavors. Gradually, in the course of long-term practice, they realized that the drugs contain all sorts of flavors, and that, therefore, they contain all kinds of different abilities. When the *Neijing* states: acrid disperses, sour contracts, sweet relaxes, bitter hardens, and salty softens, then this is an inductive classification of the effects of the five flavors. On this basis, the people of former times added (the following insights): an acrid flavor is able to disperse and to activate; a sour flavor is able to contract and to roughen; a sweet flavor is able to supplement and to harmonize; a bitter flavor is able to dry and to drain; a salty flavor is able to soften and to purge.

The associations between the five flavors and the five phases are (the following): sour belongs to wood; bitter belongs to fire; sweet belongs to soil; acrid belongs to metal; and salty belongs to water. Hence the relationships between the five flavors and the five depots are the following: sour enters the liver; bitter enters the heart; sweet enters the spleen; acrid enters the lung; and salty enters the kidneys. However, as is the case with the four qi outlined above, the nature of each of the five flavors is unilateral. It may regulate an imbalance of the qi of the depots, but it may also harm the qi of the depots and generate illness.

Text 16.7

每一种药物对于某一脏腑经络都有它的特殊作用，前人就将某一药物归入某一脏腑经络。例如麻黄入肺与膀胱二经，说明麻黄的作用主要在于肺与膀胱二经，凡是肺和膀胱感受寒邪，用麻黄的辛温来祛散最为合适。故麻黄善于治太阳病表寒，亦能止咳平喘，这种方法，叫做"归经"。归经，在实际应用上具有重要意义。如前所说，寒药能治热病，热药能治寒病，清热药多是寒凉性的，祛寒药多是温热性的，这是一个原则。但同一热症或寒症，产生的部位不同，有在表，有在里，有在脏，有在腑。比如某种寒凉药，能清表热，不一定能清里热，能清肺脏的热，不一定能清胃腑的热。于此可见，药物在人体上发挥作用，各有其适应范围，归经便是指出药物的适应范围。

Transliteration 16.7

Měi-yī zhǒng yào-wù duì-yú mǒu-yī zàng-fǔ jīng-luò dōu yǒu tā-de tè-shū zuò-yòng, qián-rén jiù jiāng mǒu-yī yào-wù guī-rù mǒu-yī zàng-fǔ jīng-luò. Lì-rú má-huáng rù fèi yǔ páng-guāng èr jīng, shuō-míng má-huáng de zuò-yòng zhǔ-yào zài-yú fèi yǔ páng-guāng èr jīng, fán-shì fèi hé páng-guāng gǎn-shòu hán-xié, yòng má-huáng de xīn-wēn lái qū sàn zuì-wéi hé-shì. Gù má-huáng shàn-yú zhì tài-yáng-bìng biǎo-hán, yì néng zhǐ ké píng-chuǎn, zhè zhǒng fāng-fǎ, jiào-zuò "guī-jīng."

Guī-jīng, zài shí-jì yìng-yòng shàng jù-yǒu zhòng-yào yì-yì. Rú-qián-suǒ-shuō, hán-yào néng zhì rè-bìng, rè-yào néng zhì hán-bìng, qīng-rè-yào duō shì hán-liáng xìng de, qū-hán-yào duō shì wēn-rè xìng de, zhè shì yī ge yuán-zé. Dàn tóng-yī rè-zhèng huò hán-zhèng, chǎn-shēng de bù-wèi bù-tóng, yǒu zài biǎo, yǒu zài lǐ, yǒu zài zàng, yǒu zài fǔ. Bǐ-rú mǒu-zhǒng hán-liáng-yào, néng qīng biǎo-rè, bù-yī-dìng néng qīng lǐ-rè, néng qīng fèi-zàng de rè, bù-yī-dìng néng qīng wèi-fǔ de rè. Yú-cǐ-kě-jiàn, yào-wù zài rén-tǐ shàng fā-huī zuò-yòng, gè yǒu qí shì-yìng-fàn-wéi, guī-jīng biàn shì zhǐ-chū yào-wù de shì-yìng-fàn-wéi.

Vocabulary 16.7

每一	měi-yī	each
归入	guī-rù	associate with
在于	zài-yú	be in; take place in
合适	hé-shì	appropriate
善于	shàn-yú	be good for; be well-suited for
归经	guī-jīng	conduit entry
如前所说	rú-qián-suǒ-shuō	as stated before
清热药	qīng-rè-yào	drugs cooling heat
祛寒药	qū-hán-yào	drugs eliminating cold
有	yǒu	some
在	zài	be there; exist
胃腑	wèi-fǔ	the stomach
指出	zhǐ-chū	point out
适应范围	shì-yìng-fàn-wéi	scope of indications

Translation 16.7

Each single drug exerts its special effect on specific conduits and network (vessels) of the depots and palaces, and the people of former times associated a specific drug with the conduit and network (vessels) of a specific depot and palace. For example, (it was concluded that) mahuang enters the two conduits of the lung and of the bladder, and this was to explain that the effects of mahuang take place mainly in the two conduits of the lung and of the bladder. Whenever the lung and the bladder are affected by cold evil, it is most appropriate to use the acrid (flavor) and the warm (qi) of mahuang to eliminate and disperse (the cold evil). Hence mahuang is well-suited for treating major yang illnesses and outside cold; it is also able to stop coughing and to calm panting. This approach is called "conduit entry."

The conduit entry is of profound significance in the actual application (of drugs). As stated before, cold drugs can cure heat illnesses, and hot drugs can cure cold illnesses. Drugs that cool heat are often of a cold-cool nature, and drugs that eliminate cold are often of a warm-hot nature. That is one principle. However, the locations where identical pathoconditions of heat or cold emerge are different; sometimes (they emerge) in the outside, sometimes in the inside; sometimes in the depots, sometimes in the palaces. For instance, a certain drug of cold-cool (nature) which is able to cool outside heat is not necessarily able to cool inside heat; it can cool the heat in the lung, but is not necessarily able to cool the heat of the stomach. That shows that all the effects exerted by a drug in the human body have their respective scope of indications; the conduit entry points out a (specific) drug's scope of indications.

一药有一药的作用，通过药与药的配合，能促使作用加强，或减少不良反应，发挥更好的效能，这是中药配合应用的重要意义。前人在实践中认识到药与药配合的反应，不仅指出了有利的一面，还指出了不良的一面。共分六类：

1. 相须：即两种功效相同的药物经过配合使用，可以互相促进加强效果。

2. 相使：两种不同功效的药物，配合后能使直达病所，发挥更好的疗效。

3. 相畏：一种药物能受到另一种药物的克制，因而减低或消除其烈性的，叫做相畏。

4. 相恶：两药合用时，因牵制而减低其效能，叫做相恶，恶是不喜欢的意思。

5. 相杀：指一种药物能消除另一种药物的毒性。

6. 相反：合用后能发生剧烈的副作用。相反和相畏的药必须慎用。

Transliteration 16.8

Yī yào yǒu yī yào de zuò-yòng, tōng-guò yào yǔ yào de pèi-hé, néng cù-shǐ zuò-yòng jiā-qiáng, huò jiǎn-shǎo bù-liáng fǎn-yìng, fā-huī gèng-hǎo de xiào-néng, zhè shì zhōng-yào pèi-hé yìng-yòng de zhòng-yào yì-yì. Qián-rén zài shí-jiàn zhōng rèn-shi-dào yào yǔ yào pèi-hé de fǎn-yìng, bù-jǐn zhǐ-chū le yǒu-lì de yī miàn, hái zhǐ-chū le bù-liáng de yī miàn. Gòng fēn liù lèi:

1.Xiāng-xū: jí liǎng zhǒng gōng-xiào xiāng-tóng de yào-wù jīng-guò pèi-hé shǐ-yòng, kě-yǐ hù-xiāng cù-jìn jiā-qiáng xiào-guǒ.

2. Xiāng-shǐ: liǎng zhǒng bù-tóng gōng-xiào de yào-wù, pèi-hé hòu néng shǐ zhí dá bìng-suǒ, fā-huī gèng-hǎo de liáo-xiào.

3. Xiāng-wèi: yī zhǒng yào-wù néng shòu-dào lìng-yī zhǒng yào-wù de kè-zhì, yīn-ér jiǎn-dī huò xiāo-chú qí liè xìng de, jiào-zuò xiāng-wèi.

4.Xiāng-wù: liǎng yào hé yòng shí, yīn qiān-zhì ér jiǎn-dī qí xiào-néng, jiào-zuò xiāng-wù, wù shì bù xǐ-huān de yì-si.

5. Xiāng-shā: zhǐ yī zhǒng yào-wù néng xiāo-chú lìng-yī zhǒng yào-wù de dú-xìng.

6. Xiāng-fǎn: hé yòng hòu néng fā-shēng jù-liè de fù-zuò-yòng. Xiāng-fǎn hé xiāng-wèi de yào bì-xū shèn yòng.

Vocabulary 16.8

配合	pèi-hé	combine
好	hǎo	good
更好	gèng-hǎo	better
相须	xiāng-xū	relationship of accentuation
促进	cù-jìn	stimulate
相使	xiāng-shǐ	relationship of stimulation
达	dá	reach
病所	bìng-suǒ	location of an illness
相畏	xiāng-wèi	relationship of awe
烈	liè	violent
相恶	xiāng-wù	relationship of aversion
牵制	qiān-zhì	restrain
喜欢	xǐ-huān	like; love
相杀	xiāng-shā	relationship of killing
剧烈	jù-liè	violent
副作用	fù-zuò-yòng	side effect

Translation 16.8

One single drug exerts its specific effects. Through combining (a specific) drug with (another specific) drug it is possible to stimulate (their) effects to become stronger, or to diminish unwanted reactions (in the patient and thereby have the drugs) display even better therapeutic effects. This is the profound significance of the combined application (of drugs) in Chinese pharmaceutics. In the course of practical experience, the people of former times recognized the responses (of the patients) to the combinations of drugs; they pointed out not only the beneficial aspects (of drug combinations), they also pointed out the negative aspects. Altogether they distinguished among six categories (of mutual effects of drugs used in combination):

1. Relationship of accentuation: That is, two drugs with similar effects are applied in combination and are able to mutally strengthen their effects.

2. Relationship of stimulation: Two drugs with different effects may stimulate (each other), after they have been combined, to proceed directly to the location of an illness and to display even better therapeutic effects.

3. Relationship of awe: If one drug is restrained (in its effects) by another drug, and if as a result its violent nature is thereby reduced or eliminated, that is called relationship of awe.

4. Relationship of aversion: If two drugs are used in combination and, as a result, (mutually) restrain or diminish their effects, that is called relationship of aversion.

5. Relationship of killing: This refers to (the fact that) one drug can eliminate the toxic nature of another drug.

6. Relationship of clashing: After being applied in combinations, (drugs) may develop violent side effects.

Drugs that are in a relationship of clashing or of awe must be used with caution.